HEALING PLANTS
VOLUME II

HEALING PLANTS

Insights Through Spiritual Science

Volume II

Wilhelm Pelikan

Illustrated by Walther Roggenkamp

Published by the Medical Section of the School for Spiritual Science
at the Goetheanum, Dornach, Switzerland

English by Harold Jurgens and Gerald Karnow MD

MERCURY PRESS

Original title:
Heilpflanzenkunde
Der Mensch und die Heilpflanzen
Band II
Wilhelm Pelikan
Mit Pflanzenzeichnungen von Walther Roggenkamp
Herausgegeben von der medizinischen Sektion der freien Hochschule
für
Geisteswissenschaft am Goetheanum
Philosophisch-Anthroposophischer Verlag Goetheanum/Dornach
(Switzerland)

Copyright © 2012 of this translation
by Mercury Press

Cover art and design by Jorge Sanz Cardona
ISBN 978-1-957569-31-4

Published in the USA by:

Mercury Press
an imprint of SteinerBooks
PO Box 58
Hudson, NY 12534

www.steinerbooks.org

Contents

Editor's Preface i

The Author's Preface to Volume II of Healing Plants ii

Preface to the First 1957 Edition iii

Concerning the Illustrations in this Book v

Medicinal Herbs from the Lower Plant Kingdom 7

Algae— Phycophyta 8

Fungi — Mycetophyta 11

Lichens 14

Ferns – Filicinae 16

Horsetails – Equisetinae 24

Medicinal Plants from the Upper Plant Kingdom 25

Evergreen Trees and Shrubs – Coniferae 25

The Pine Family – Pinaceae 30

Cypress–like Shrubs and Trees – Cypressaceae 33

St. John's Worts – Guttiferae 37

Rock foil plants – Saxifragaceae: *Silica Process, Limestone and Light Processes* 43

Thick leafed plants – Crassulaceae 47

The Gourds – Cucurbitaceae 52

Irises – Iridaceae 60

Grasses – Gramineae 66

Arums – Araceae: *Flowering Processes in the Root Region* 82

Catkin Bearers – Amentiflorae 89

Willows – Salicaceae: Salicin and Tannin Process 100

Rues – Rutaceae: *The Masters of Tropical Warmth Processes* 107

Pinks – Caryophyllaceae – Chickweeds, Stitchworts, Campions ... 116

Grape Family – Vitaceae 119

Honeysuckles – Caprifoliaceae 126

Sea Buckthorn – Hippophae rhamnoides: *Images of a Plant's Essential Nature and Therapeutic Imaginations* 130

Vitamins 137

The Totality of Food Plants 143

The Extra Corporeal "Organs" of Plants 145

The Nitrogen, Oxygen, Carbon and Hydrogen Organs in the Atmosphere 155

Myrtles – Myrtaceae: *Fruit and Spice Plants* 163

Crane bills – Geraniaceae 168

Wood Sorrels – Oxalidaceae: *The Oxalic Acid Process in Plant and Man* 170

Mallows – Malvaceae: *The Formation of Mucilage and Fibers* 178

Snapdragons - Scrophulariaceae 182

Bindweeds – Convolvulaceae 198

The Olive Family – Oleaceae: *The Process that Forms Oils in the Plant Kingdom* 200

The Dogbane Family - Apocynaceae 209

The Heather Family – Ericaceae: *Northern Fruits* 216

Primroses – Primulaceae: *Plants with Etheric Vernal Rhythms* 224

Medicinal Plants for the Liver 237

Medicinal Plants for the Kidneys 244

Medicinal Plants for the Lungs 252

Medicinal Plants for the Heart 257

Index of Illustrations 261

Subject index 263

Editor's Preface

With this second volume of his Healing Plants Wilhelm Pelikan rounds off the first volume that was published four years ago into a comprehensive and modern descriptive work on medicinal plants. The foundations and the methods used have remained the same. Rudolf Steiner's spiritual investigations are the firm foundation on which the far reaching structure is base and the style that is raised into the imaginative realm and that lets a large number of new medicinal plant entities arise before us is used with the same mastery as before.

The present volume's contents considerably supplement the list of plants already described. A number of medicinal plants from the least developed end of the plant kingdom are presented right at the beginning. Rudolf Steiner gives a number of indications about them, and they have proven to be quite useful in therapy. Two groups stand out as particularly good examples of Pelikan's skill in presenting things in the first third of the book. The grasses and grains whose study is of the greatest interest for an understanding of human nutrition, and then later on trees and shrubs – especially those which have catkins, for their division into seven kinds gives one an inkling of how they can be assigned to processes of disease and healing in man.

Pelikan's sketch of Sea Buckthorn's (Hippophae rhamnoides) essential nature is an outstanding example of the independent way in which he works with his subject matter. Rudolf Steiner did not say anything about this plant, but Pelikan treats it in such a way that one can immediately see its value for human health. That is particularly important for the method with which anthroposophic medical personnel wants to establish its applications.

Therefore the present volume can also be sent out into the world with joy and satisfaction at the successful way that it turned out. It will give the hopefully numerous readers impressive new insights into the primal relation between plant and man.

Gerhard Schmidt

The Author's Preface to Volume II of Healing Plants

When my first volume of Healing Plants was published a few years ago, I already had plenty of material for another volume, which only had to receive its final form. However, it was still uncertain how many readers would be interested in one volume, let alone two. This question has now been answered. A surprisingly large interest in the nature of medicinal plants became manifest. One half of the first edition sold out in a short time and a lively exchange of ideas with many readers developed.

This encouraged me to dare to complete and publish the present volume, although one really should read Volume I first. Herewith a certain rounding off of the field that was presented has been attained and a large number of new medicinal plants appear before the reader. Volume I could help open an organ of perception for the peculiar fact that plants are not only a source of food but also of healing. With this opened organ one will take a joyful look at the large number of plants that are presented here. Already the sight of the inexhaustible wealth of salutary nature can have a rejuvenating, healing effect upon a person.

This work could not have been finished or even begun if the lifework of that great man who knew nature and the spirit and whose birthday is being celebrated for the hundredth time this year – Rudolf Steiner – was not readily accessible to everyone. I would like to thank him first of all, and then also the School for Spiritual Science at the Goetheanum, and especially its Medical Section, which has also given its support to the present volume. My thanks go out to all friends who have helped me with advice, work, suggestions for improvements, supportive interest and corrections. I am very glad that I had Walther Roggenkamp, the illustrator at my side again for this second volume. For what would plant descriptions be without expressive pictures! I thank the publishers for their usual careful and thorough production. I also have warm thoughts for all those who worked energetically in this field before me, and I especially hope for successors who will do much more than what has been attained so far. For all life wants a higher life.

What will such future achievements be like? Courageous thinkers make well founded guesses about that.

Wilhelm Pelikan,
May 1967

Preface to the First 1957 Edition

The ancient's medicine was largely based upon plants. Interest in the latter were pushed in to the background by advances in analytic and synthetic chemistry and by the pharmacology that worked hand in hand with it in the 19th century, but the interest of professional scientists is being directed towards them again due to the discovery of antibiotics and to the investigation of strong drugs like those in crataegus, licorice, amni visnaga and rauwolfia. One could speak of a renaissance of medicinal botany if it weren't for the strong probability that investigators will continue to work in the same old ruts toward an isolation of "active ingredients," an investigation of their chemical structures, and artificial syntheses along the lines of chemistry.

However, one can speak of a new birth of medicinal botany, since a medicine that has been extended by modern spiritual investigations (Anthroposophy) can point to new essential relations between plant and man. Such a medicinal botany can be called rational in the real sense of the word, for it is based on descriptions of plants and human beings that can relate to each other in an exact way. In one's striving for knowledge it becomes possible to project man into all the plants, and the plant into man. For such a way of knowing, sick human nature or the totality of all pathological processes finds its counter-world, reflection and phyto-projection in the realm of medicinal plants. It is the task of the present book to outline this. The author is quite aware that this attempt is filled with his personal defects – but he dared to make it since so many results of Rudolf Steiner's investigations are available.

The present descriptions on the results of work with plants, which was begun in small groups in 1921 through an elaboration of Goethe's theory of metamorphosis, was continued through the encouragement of Eugene Kolisko's genial personality, and strongly promoted by the books and lectures of the well-known botanist A. Usteri. The decisive steps towards a medicinal botany in the sense meant here proceeded from lectures which Rudolf Steiner gave to physicians. A working circle of doctors, pharmacists and chemists in Stuttgart that formed in connection with one of these series of lectures can be looked upon as the source of the germinal ideas in this book.

These germinal ideas received an important impulse for their further development from the papers and books of Gunther Wachsmuth, especially from his book *The Etheric Formative Forces in the Cosmos, Earth and Man*. This was followed by the fundamental descriptions of the trailblazing botanist and teacher, Gerbert Grohman for the founding of a spiritual scientific botany. One should also mention numerous studies on medicinal plants by Weleda personnel which have been published in the Weleda Journal and various other places for almost thirty years now. More recently we have Werner Simonis' thorough "medical–botanical descriptions of the essential nature of individual medicinal plants," who has written over 40 monographs on the latter. There are also a number of subtle studies on medicinal herbs in the professional, anthroposophic, medical literature.

However, someone still had to give a systematic, overall presentation of medicinal plants. May you readers kindly take the present book as a contribution towards this end.

In conclusion the author gladly fulfills his duty of thanking all the people who have helped him with his work, and he gives special thanks to his first botany teacher, his dear wife, without whose many sided help this book would never have been written.

Wilhelm Pelikan, 1957

Concerning the Illustrations in this Book

The reader will find that the explanations about particularly important medicinal herbs are accompanied by the attempts of our artist to illustrate what can never be made sufficiently clear through words. The characteristic, essential features of the particular plant are supposed to come out through the play of black and white and through the dynamics of the lines and planes in these pictures. No attempt has been made to give naturalistically accurate pictures. One can recognize the represented plants, but this recognition is not based on an imitation of the outer phenomenon, especially where the picture becomes a vignette or signature of the text. The laws of the graphic arts have their own way of reproducing the plant that has been created by the laws of nature outside. Thereby something can become visible which is not shown or is at most indicated by a mere look at Nature and which only appears to the eye of the spirit. The artist's work reveals what Nature conceals.

MEDICINAL HERBS FROM THE LOWER PLANT KINGDOM

ALGAE, FUNGI, LICHENS, FERNS, HORSETAILS

"Perfect" plants are flowering plants, for they bring the essential nature of plants, the idea of "plantkind" or Goethe's archetypal plant, to expression most perfectly. Although they appeared last in the course of plantkind's evolution, this evolution aimed in their direction right from the start. We must look upon the urge of plantkind to disclose its essential nature completely, as the driving force behind this evolution. It became a developmental force before it became manifest as sensory forms.

Take a perfect plant with its roots, shoot, leaves, flowers and fruits. It reveals itself in its quite particular position in terrestrial creation in the kingdoms of nature, and in the forces and elements of terrestrial existence. Through its division into root, shoot, leaf, flower it shows how it is standing as a totality within the more comprehensive whole of all earth existence, whose summary and leitmotif is the human being. It is a mediating entity between earth and the cosmos, dark and light, and also between the mineral and animal kingdoms. Since the plant has brought its essential nature into a sensory, phenomenal form to such an extent, it will not be able to develop appreciably beyond its present state, unless a new creative impulse takes hold of the entire earth existence. But that would involve an entirely new creation. This will someday occur, just as the present creation of the earth proceeded from previous creations. One can read about this in many of Rudolf Steiner's books and lectures, as for instance, in his *Occult Science, an Outline*.

Thus, present day flowering plants are finished to a large extent, and their spiritual element has become visible to the senses. The so–called lower plants are imperfect from this point of view; they are preliminary manifestations of present–day plants in this or that direction, and this gives them a one–sided appearance. One can derive them from fully developed plants in one's imagination by suppressing some of the plants' forces, whereby other forces become predominant. A horsetail, equisetum arvense, is really only a stem, a fern is only a leaf, algae are only onflowing stem and leaf formations, a fungus is a "root blossom" (Grohmann coined this apt word) which relinquished the formation of leaves, and it needs the rotting leaves of other, more perfect plants. Molds, rusts and mildews get no further than the unicellular stage and have completely renounced any real form of their own. A "complete plant" only displays this condition temporarily, as for instance when it forms pollen cells and scatters them like dust. Such primitive plant formations have no overall shapes. Nevertheless they can't really do without the latter. They have to connect themselves with foreign totalities. This is where we get into the broad realm of the parasitism.

However, another impulse works into this whole, large realm of still imperfect plants where the formative impulses of the archetypal plant are still floating above them more than they are permeating them. This impulse comes out of the world's past. The reader has already run into the description of world evolution that is given by anthroposophic spiritual science several times in this medicinal botany. It tells us about previous stages of the present earthly creation and we will mainly be interested in the ancient Moon creation here. This produced three kingdoms of nature which were in between our present day kingdoms — a plant mineral kingdom between our present mineral and plant kingdoms, an animal–plant kingdom between the present plant and animal kingdoms, and a highest kingdom between the present animals and men that contained our ancestors. There are plenty of reminders of the old animal–plants among our present plants, and we have mentioned many of them in volume 1 of this work, as in the section on Flesh–Digesting Plants, the section on Poppies, etc. This past also enables one to understand the close connections between plants and animals, the way they are created for each other as for instance, flowers and their visitors, gall formations and many other things. Of course one also has connections in the oldest, lower plants, so that the boundary between plants and lower animals is not very distinct.

*

ALGAE— PHYCOPHYTA

It would take too much space to even give an overview of the 8,000 or so species of algae that have been found to date. We will only try to pick out some typical things in order to become aware of their curative connections with human beings.

The algae's life sphere is illumined water. They give its streaming, flowing, dripping and reuniting, atomizing and regrouping nature a kind of a living form. The largest kinds and most of them populate the oceans, but strands of algae float around on the floor of every brook, in every pond and marshy pool. Species of algae congregate on the bottoms of springs, on damp parts of fields, moist leaves, tree trunks and other surfaces, inside clams, snails, sponges and worms and in the furs of sloths, and even glaciers and the snow fields of high mountains and the polar regions have their algae. Just as water can be individual drops, streaming threads or spreading sheets, so there are unicellular, stringy algae which flow together into colonies and take on the forms of higher plants with stems and leaves, floating branched shrubs and even treelike formations. The formation of green leaf pigment makes them all true plants, but ones for whom only water (that has air dissolved in it) and light exist into its terrestrial existence – dampness and light – but not solid, mineral earth. For they are unable to form roots or the flowers that produce fruits. The algae proceeded from a creative, archetypal plant during an old condition of our planet when there was as yet no solid earth. Rudolf Steiner called this stage of development the Lemurian epoch, and he spoke about the vitalized atmosphere at that time, which had the consistency of very dilute egg white, in which cloudlike plant formations swam or floated, and became green or lost their green depending on their biological rhythms. The paintings on the large cupola of the first Goetheanum included one on Lemuria. There one can see gigantic algae formations or seaweed that flowed through a mobile, fiery element.

Algae were the first true plants, which found their havens in the earth's waters, and which retained something from the time they were first created, when earth evolution strove towards the formation of solid core in the earth and therewith all conditions changed. Algae are true plants and they live from and with light. Blue, green, brown and red algae form, depending on the depth of the water and on how much light there is in it, the latter kinds are in deep water where the light is dim. They assimilate carbon dioxide and the necessary salts from the water with great force; they exhale the oxygen they form – sometimes in the bladder–like formations they carry on the water's surface. They condense the very dilute mineral components in them into siliceous, calcareous inclusions, into considerable amounts of iodine, etc., so that the ashes of certain algae used to be an important source of iodine. There are no poisonous algae and the protein and carbohydrate content of some algae make them into important foods.

Rudolf Steiner tells us why algae can be used as medicinal plants. Algae are plants without strongly developed roots or flowers. The flower and root are actually pushed together. The leaves are their main organ which produces everything else. The leaf predominates, so that there is no intensive relation to the earth in these plants. There is also no intensive relation to the outer cosmos, but only a relation to everything that occurs in the watery and airiform element directly at the earth's surface. Algae are plants that are entirely immersed in the interactions between air and the watery element. Now the peculiar thing is that these plants exert a very strong attraction on the very small quantities of sulfur that are distributed everywhere in water and air. Thereby these plants, if introduced into the rhythmic system, are particularly suitable for establishing a harmony between the astral body and the etheric body.[1] One can resort to the use of algae as remedies if this harmony is disrupted because the physical and etheric bodies refuse to let the astral body enter them sufficiently. Such a remedy attracts the healthy astrality in the world, for algae pull in the astrality from the surrounding air. (On the other hand, one can use fungi as a remedy if the insufficient care of the physical and etheric bodies by the forces of the astral body comes from the fact that the I organization makes too great demands upon the astral body and does not let it get into the etheric body.)

Rudolf Steiner recommended the use of algae preparations for young patients who had the constitution described above, and also for diseases that temporarily produces similar relations between man's members, as in scarlet fever, for example. An important developmental task of growing children is to adapt the body that they got from their parents in such a way that it can be used as an instrument by the spiritual being that has come down from the spiritual world. This does not happen without a struggle; children's diseases are an expression of these struggles. If this battle is raged by a strong, energetic individuality, one can have the dramatic outcome of a bout with scarlet fever, where the main thing is to let the transformative intervention of the patient's higher members into the inherited body occur in a controlled way, where this inherited body is tuned in such a way that it opens itself to this intervention in the right way. If one uses algae as a remedy the vehemence of this battle is reduced and the doctor gains control over its course.

---

[1] See Volume I for the conceptual content of and the justification for the use of these terms.

Fungi — Mycetophyta

Again it is impossible to even name the great number of fungus species here, tens of thousands of them are known and many geographical regions have not even been investigated very thoroughly yet; we will have to limit ourselves to a group of the type and to an investigation of the healing possibilities. In contrast to the algae, which permeate the earth's illuminated waters with green life, fungi like dark, moist earth that is sometimes warmed through by molds, although they also do well in the coldest regions. The earth that they do well in is not one that is solid and mineral but a half living realm that is filled with biological remnants and that has a lot of decomposing plant and animal matter in it; in short, it is an earth that is similar to the lowest kingdom of nature on the Old Moon, a mineral–plant realm. When one observes how fungi unfold their proliferating biological processes in the earth one is reminded of conditions on the Old Moon. The solar aspect of plants is completely suppressed in fungi; they have no leaves or green pigments. Thereby even the most highly developed fungi do not look much like plants. In addition to the fact that they like a semi-enlivened soil that is somewhat in between plants and minerals, they also have plant–animal tendencies. Protein processes are more and carbohydrate processes are less active in them than in normal plants. One finds chitinous substances in them like those in insect shells, and also other substances that are related to animals. The most primitive forms contain simple tubular cells, whereas in the highest forms the cells group together into filaments and then into masses of mycelia, which, root–like, branch out in their substrata and can combine into skins, pads or into bodies that resemble trunks or clubs, that can condense into wood–like or hornlike bodies, and which bear fruiting bodies that form the spores with which the collected, dense materials are dispersed again. The spores grow into new mycelia and mycelic bodies.

If one looks at the most perfect fungi which for instance, laymen call field mushroom, honey mushroom, fly agaric and agaric, and if one thinks of their undifferentiated structures and fused filaments, one gets the feeling that their forms have been stamped on them from outside rather than developed from within. If one looks to see where one can find models for such forms in normal plants one finds root filaments and tree stumps, which however pass over into something like blossoms here, as one sees in the rods and clubs of certain arums, which can have Boeletus mushroom like forms. (See the chapter on arums in this book) These upper formations conceal sporangia and spores. Thus the "root blossom" term that Grohmann coined hits the nail on the head. Root processes and flower processes push into each other to the exclusion of any rhythmic system in between; no green leaves appear.

This is why fungi have placed themselves on the degradative side of Nature; they live on disintegrating life or on life that has been abandoned by its formative forces, which would otherwise lead to trillions of mummified formations, and would fill the earth with layers of biological remnants that would pile up into geological formations. Thus fungi are saprophytes that live on decaying or dead plants, or they are parasites that are not completely controlled by their formative forces. They feed on anything that has been shed or has fallen off, such as fruits, leaves, bark, wood, hair, feathers and horns; every plant species and every part of one has its specific parasitic fungus which simply belongs to it. The attacks of some of them have a strong effect on the host's system of formative forces, and they call forth metamorphic forces that respond by generating so-called witch's brooms and galls. This shows the astralized nature of fungi that is related to animals; it is something similar to what gall wasps and gnats do when they prick leaves and lay their eggs. (See the section here on rye grass and ergot under Grains.)

Fermenting, rusting and molding occurs through them; they destroy the shapes of things that were once alive. So it is not surprising that they seem to have such imperfect shapes. One order, the Entomophthorales, attacks insects and brings death and destruction into the realm of caterpillars, flies, etc. The point of attack for this is given by the insects' formative forces that tend towards rigidification.

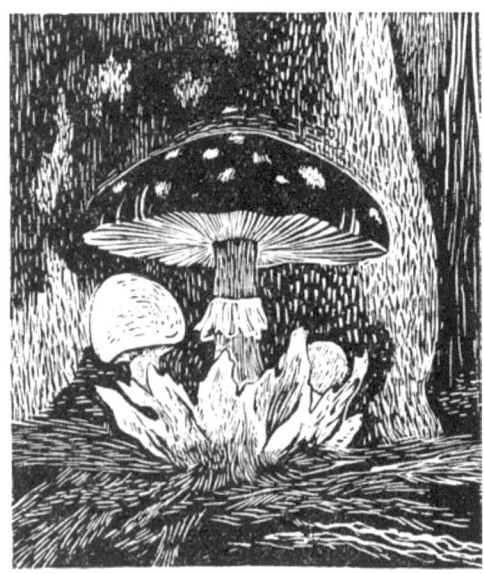

Rudolf Steiner recommended the use of certain poisonous and nonpoisonous mushrooms as remedies. When he spoke about the use of algae he also said that one can use mushrooms as remedies for disorders that are caused when the I organization makes excessive demand upon the astral body and does not let it enter the etheric body; these plants attract the astral forces in their environment very strongly.

One will see that Nature illustrates what was said above if one observes how plants which pull their flower nature deep down into their root region, like the arums which we have often mentioned and the Aristoloceraceae, etc. begin to look very much like mushrooms, when they choose dark growing places and thereby strongly suppress their leaf nature, or when they suppress it completely as in the case of certain root parasites (Hydroraceae) and flower parasites (Rafflesiaceae). For here one can see that astrality has been powerfully attracted by the root region.

This attraction is too strong in the case of mushroom poisoning, and the far reaching degradative and destructive phenomena in the victim's organs, which are somewhat similar to phosphorus poisoning, are the result of this overly strong intervention.

Thus fungi tend to work upon the upper man and his nervous system, which feeds on the overall organism in a "parasitic" way, and which has a degradative function that is similar to that of fungi in the overall nature process. Fungi are "root blossoms" and as such they will stimulate the metabolic system in the brain and nerves and thereby be able to bring about anabolic processes in a nervous system that has been injured through certain diseases, where one has brain flu, palsy, etc. According to Rudolf Steiner poisonous mushrooms that have been pharmaceutically prepared in the right way can help tissues to regenerate themselves. Even though this applies mainly to nerve tissue, this regenerative effect can also be carried into other organ regions by combining them with other substances, as for instance, into the skeletal systems. Steiner recommended a preparation made of Agaricus muscaria, fern spores, calcium carbonate, silver and phosphorus, for osteomalacia, where the bones lose their formative forces through a chaotization of their calcium process (osteoporosis).

Other fungi that Rudolf Steiner recommended as remedies, were Conthorellus ciborius, Psolliota compestris, Amanita caesarea, Merulius lacrimans and a fungus that grows on evergreen trees.

Lichens

The lichens[2] provide a number of good remedies, and Rudolf Steiner gave some new indications for their use. They represent an important evolutionary form of plants on earth, for in the lichens the plant kingdom came down to the solid mineral earth, whereas the algae were at home in a sunny "watery earth", and fungi lived in a dark, "Moon earth". Botanists speak of a symbiosis between fungi and algae, where the fungus process took the algae nature into itself in the formation of lichens. The lichens were extremely tough, biologically speaking, and they seem to have no restrictions as to where they can live. They cover bare rocks, proliferate on wood and bark, take over areas in the polar zones and high up in the mountains, and they enable animals and man to stay in places where they would otherwise not be able to live. They are the vegetables in the tundras, they appear in the far north as earth lichens, whereas they become tree and bark lichens towards the warmer zones, especially in foggy, moist forests on mountains. Here one can see again that trees are really a protrusion of the earth. The turf of lichens is tree bark in the tropics, the ground in the far north, and both of these in the temperate zones. Icelandic moss, reindeer moss, manna lichens (the Kirgiz's earthbread) are life saving earth lichens of the north; Beard moss (Usnea barbata) can represent the branch lichens of the central European mountain forests; tree scratcher (Evernia prunastri) the deciduous tree mosses; cup moss, circle moss and nap moss, the rock mosses.

The forms which lichens can take on range from powdery indications, crustaceous growths, skinlike or gelatinous coverings up to something like leaves, and finally to stemmed, bushy protrusions or cartilaginous-leafed, curly cramped shapes that seem to be made out of cardboard, or tough, leathery substances. The common name "curly-cramps tea" for the dried lichen leaves gives one a good idea of what they look like. Thus the most highly developed lichens have everything like a normal plant form — at least outwardly.

When minerals were pushed down out of the living earth during the Lemurian epoch, only the toughest life could accompany them, plants

---

[2] See W. C. Simonis's excellent description of lichens in his *Die unbekannte Heilpflanze*

that were connected with a formative force that is known as life ether.[3] Only a plant that is particularly hardy can live in the dying bark which some plants eject out into the dead mineral environment, at least, it has to be hardier than the plant which is expelling bark and which is no longer sending any life into the bark forming process. The material, physical world and the etheric, formative forces correspond to each other: physical warmth to warmth ether, air to light ether, water and other fluids to the chemical or sound ether, and solids to the life ether, which Rudolf Steiner also called the meaning ether. (Just as solids can hold fluids and can give them a particular form as their vessel so life ether gives chemical ether a meaningful, individual form. The chemism of an organism is distinguished from chemical processes in the dead, mineral realm by the meaningful form that is individually adapted to life as a whole. The chemical ether in the transformation of substances and the anabolism of an organism is permeated and formed by life ether in a meaningful way.) Lichens live in places where life passes over into lifelessness and living chemism glides off into the chemistry of dead materials, and they maintain themselves there through a particularly strong development of life ether forces.

This can also be seen in the "lichen chemistry" that is really quite complicated for such primitive plants. The excretion of large amounts of lichenous acids is able to disintegrate limestone, schist and granite substrata to a large extent and thereby open them up to biological activity. Thus the life of lichens is a counter process to the earth's mineralization. Lichens protect themselves against lignification processes through the development of large quantities of mucilage. Some lichens form intense yellow, red, violet or blue dyes. Litmus is the best known of these, and its change from purple into red or blue tells chemistry students whether a solution is acidic or alkaline.

The development of lungs only became possible with the appearance of solid earth and continents, the separation of the waters, and the contact of land and the moist atmosphere. Thereby they have a

---

[3] Life ether, chemical or sound ether, light ether and warmth ether are the various existential forms of the etheric or formative force world, just as solids, fluids, gases and warmth are the forms in which things exist in the physical world. For more about this see Rudolf Steiner's *Occult Science, an Outline*, and Guenther Wachsmuth's *The Etheric Formative Forces in the Cosmos, Earth and Man*.

special connection with solids and therefore with the life ether. For further details we refer you to Rudolf Steiner's discussion about this in the *Pastoral Medicine Course*. (Also see the section on medicinal plants for the lungs at the end of this book.)

The guidelines for the use of lichens as remedies

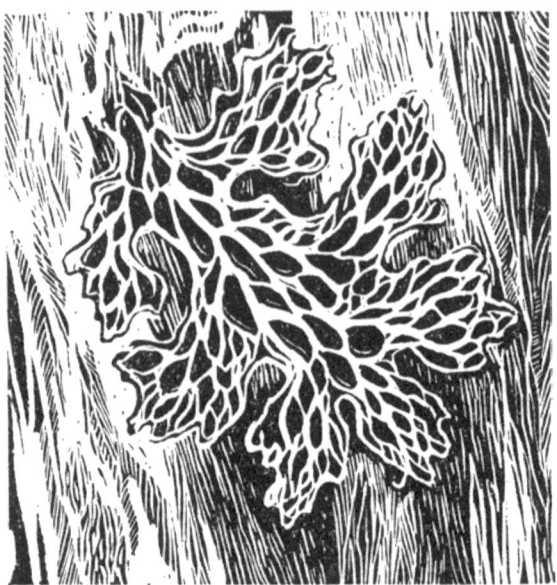

proceed from these connections. They are good for treating certain lung diseases and they counteract general asthenia and lowered vitality. Rudolf Steiner recommended lichen preparations combined with other plants as injections, baths and teas for such conditions, and also for the support of mistletoe therapy for cancer.

FERNS – FILICINAE

Whereas we have experienced preliminary stages in the manifestation of plants upon the earth in our study of algae, fungi and lichens that are reminiscent of Old Moon evolution and Old Sun evolution, the plant element appears in Pteridophytes, the ferns, horsetails and club mosses, in forms in which even an open-minded person– not just a botanist – can see the "real plants of our earth."

For the primal organ of all plants – the green leaf – is the main organ for the first time in the true forms that we will look at next and right away with the greatest possible development of form that one could imagine. In ferns one can see all the leaf formations that the archetypal plant could possibly invent. Leaves that are rounded, longish, narrow as grasses, smooth edged, sinuses, wavy, indented, divided in every possible way, singly, doubly, triply pinnate – it is as if the creative being in this kingdom of nature had directed all of its inventive ideas towards this one organ.

In the realm of lower plants, ferns are the first to have roots, and so they are properly connected with the mineral earth. Also we arrive at the formation of the tree here for the first time in the evolution of the plant kingdom, even though fern trees are strange phenomena, and they clearly show that a tree is really a kind of a protruding earth. In most ferns the stem formation is kept underground as a rhizome. Even in tree ferns with

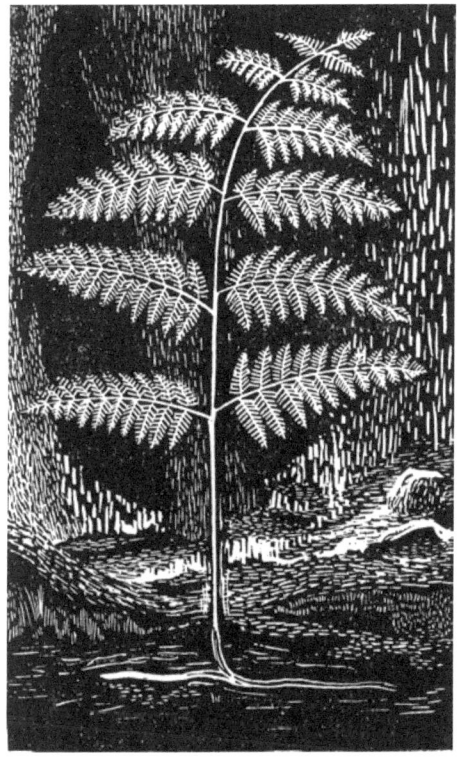

trunks as thick as a man's arm, the accessory roots that often cover them show that one is really dealing with upright rhizomes, where a funnel of green fronds sits at the upper end like a rosette just as in our woodferns on the ground.

Thus the leaf is a fern's main organ; it has force impulses in it, which the leaves of higher plants have passed on to other organs. For instance, all parts of it can continue to grow and if the tips of some ferns touch the ground, they can grow roots and form new ferns (wandering leaf). Normal plants only have such strong growth forces in their shoots. The concealed sprouting forces of the outwardly missing shoot are present in each fern leaf in an invisible way. The spiral tendency in the rhythmical arrangement of the leaves, around the stalk of higher plants, is also built into a fern leaf, and it becomes manifest in the characteristic unfurling of their fronds, which is reminiscent of an uncurling elephant's trunk. The unrestrained, shooting vitality of a fern leaf also comes to expression in the capacity of some species to form a new shoot or frond out of the surface or the ends of leaves or out of the palm's base. One finds glands that excrete sugars in others, as if they were organs on blossoms. Each fern leaf is a reproductive organ through its peculiar formation of spores. Thus it combines the functions of a root, shoot and flower, albeit in a strange way. For whereas the formation of ferns may look like an important step forward in evolution out of the realm of lower plants towards normal, present-day plants with their flowers and fruits, the formation of spores and what results is a step backwards into the realm of fungi and mosses.

For after the biological process of fern plants to have expanded into impressive leaf formations, it withdraws and produces tiny, separate cells in the formation of spores. Anyone who looks with an open mind at the clumps of spores that are arranged and ensheathed in a variety of ways on the underside of the leaves of individual species of ferns, is immediately reminded of the sporangia of many parasitic rust fungi that develop on many leaves of higher plants, except that the rusts are less developed and foreign to the plants they are sitting on, whereas the ferns bring them forth from within, out of their own nature. This impression is reinforced when the contraction into sporangia is followed by a great expansion and a dusting out into the air, whereby each spore sinks into a dark and moist place and germinates into a scale like liverwort about the size of a small fingernail, the so–called prothallium, or the kind of formation that really belongs to the next lower class of plants. On the other hand, this prothallium is a "fern blossom," for this contracted formation produces what one can compare with the anthers and pistils of higher plants, namely, archegonia and antheridia, where the latter discharge spermatozoa which move through the watery substrata towards the archegonia or egg cells and fertilize them. Then a new fern can grow out of the prothallium.

Thus what we ordinarily look upon as a fern is only the vegetative half of its existence; it pushes its other half, its flower process, the so–called bisexual phase away from it and lets it develop at another place that is separated from it. It thereby falls back to the fungi stage (the prothallia in some ferns live in the ground in a saprophytic, fungal way). Therewith the fern is continually ejecting the animal form that is reminiscent of the animal plants on the Old Moon. It purifies its plant element of the astral, animal element that the other lower plants have in them. This is why it can devote itself so completely to the formation of leaves.

There is no doubt that some ferns develop substances in their rhizomes and to a lesser extent in their leaves which prove to be very poisonous for intestinal parasites such as tape worms. One could almost call a tape worm a vegetative animal, for it sends out one node after another from the head in an almost endless vegetative process. A plant that is continually getting rid of its animal tendencies proves to be toxic towards a plant animal that lives in the intestines, or in the most plantlike region of the gastrointestinal tract. We will have to go into the connection between ferns and the digestive system in more detail when we describe the healing effects of ferns.

We must look upon ferns as a very old class of plants that is reminiscent of earth conditions in the far distant past. They reached the high point in their evolution a long time ago. Many fern species have been extinct for ages, and only their imprints are still present in coal deposits, etc., for ferns were very active in the carboniferous period. Their particular relation to water and light and the other characteristics go back to this period.

We already mentioned that most ferns love water and especially need to have enough of it in the air. That is why they frequent woods because the latter always have damp humus and a damper atmosphere than most places. Ferns also love dim light or shadows. That is why they make such good houseplants and it is another reason why ferns prefer woods. Ferns can develop best in wooded valleys with streams running through them; the waterfalls in such places with their spray support the growth of the beautiful Hart's Tongue and other rare ferns.

Thus ferns seem to have been made for a long past world with an atmosphere that was filled with water vapors and permeated by dim light. Modern spiritual investigations speak of such a stage of earth evolution, of Atlantis, of a world before Noah that came to an end through a catastrophic deluge. After that the sunlight could go through the cleared atmosphere and to the ground unhindered, and the first rainbow appeared (see Rudolf Steiner's *Occult Science, an Outline* and his *Cosmic Memory*) The appearance of the ferns must be placed at the transition between the Lemurian epoch and the Atlantean epoch, and they flourished best under foggy, Atlantean conditions. Quite a few ferns grow as epiphytes in the tropics, in which case they exist more like they did on Old Moon and they flee from mineral soil and live as nest ferns on live tree branches and trunks in the forest. New Zealand is a real fern isle which has a large number of interesting and rare kinds such as lovely tree ferns, and it also has large areas similar to the heathers in Northern Germany that are covered with bracken like the 10 foot high Pteridium esculentum. Their starchy roots used to be an important food for the Maoris.

Ferns generally avoid steppes, deserts and dry landscapes that are flooded with light and warmth. Moist cold does not hurt them for one can find them up to the edges of the glaciers in the New Zealand mountains, up to 12,000 feet high in Asia, and also high up in European and American mountains.

*

Higher, flowering plants grow from below upwards; the development of many leaves is followed by vigorous metamorphic processes. The mighty unfolding and spreading out of green leaves is followed by a contraction, a dampening down of biological forces, a simplification of forms and finally by a loss of green pigments; what was attained previously is sacrificed so that it can arise again at a higher level as a colored blossom. Thereby the plant enters the realm of air (it can now develop aromas), light, colorfulness and insects, which are connected with the flowers in a very sympathetic way. An inner process transforms the plant's nature to such an extent that it turns towards the next higher world above it, the astral or soul world, out of its own etheric formative forces. Thereby these inner processes are followed by an outer meeting with the butterflies, bees, flies, gnats, humming birds, sugar birds and even bats in the air.

A fern does not develop from a leaf upwards to higher organs; its metamorphic direction is from above downwards into the moist earth. It does not develop a sympathy for animals in the air, it develops an antipathy for the animal–plants that live like parasites in moist darkness. What results from this descent cannot emit aromas and cannot have bright colors. The flowering plants ascend from the etheric into the astral realm. In ferns an astrality sinks down into the etheric plant sphere, takes hold of fern leaves and gives them flowering properties, and also makes them slightly toxic, and it eventually pushes the fern's flower or prothallium down into the dark, damp earth.

*

A fern is unable to produce real flowers, the green leaf is the highest organ it is able to make. However, its formative gestures point to something like a prophecy of the flower form. Male fern and other species group their fronds into a funnel shaped formation. Somewhat simpler to the way that many individual leaves assemble in the development of flowers in the higher plants. Such ferns are closer to the astral principle that brings about the metamorphosis of leaves into flowers than the rhizomesof bracken (pteridium esculentum) that creep along for several yards underground and push up single shoots in a long line. The etheric principle is more active in bracken than in male fern (Filix-mas), where the astral principle is more active.

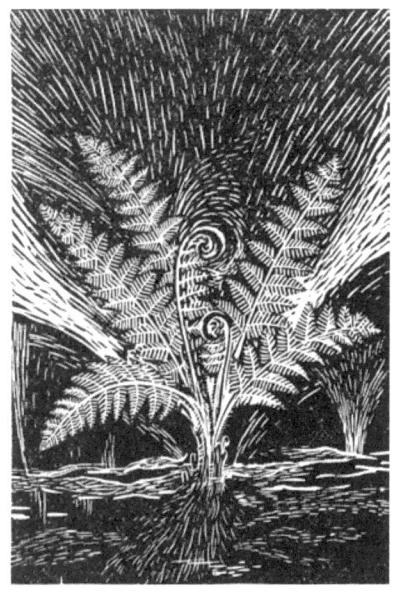

*

What one can learn from fern chemistry is added to what is expressed about the nature of ferns through their transformations. Here one finds tanning agents, fatty oils, some essential oils, filmaroon, filicine and other anti–helminthic phloroglucine derivatives. The rhizomes store starch. Investigations recently discovered an "anti–vitamin" in fern leaves, a substance that cancels the effect of thiamine or Vitamin B_1. A deficiency in the latter prevents man's higher members from properly breaking down sugar in the muscles and nervous system. This process stops at the succinic or lactic acid stage and leads to over-acidification and to injury of the tissues concerned, and therewith to serious diseases. Cattle which eat a lot of ferns get sick. Vitamin B_1 is present in plants wherever stored carbohydrates are to be taken back into the stream of life through catabolism and transformation. The shells of starchy grain seeds contain a lot of it, and so does parasitic yeast, which promotes fermentation and lives on the saccharine substrata that are provided for it by substances that have accumulated from the fruit processes of the plants. The anti-vitamin in ferns inhibits such processes.

This may be connected with the fact that the ferns have a certain capacity to inhibit decomposition. If one investigates a fern rhizome one can still see the leaf base armor of previous years that cover the new shoots with earthy brown. Foods wrapped in fern leaves stay fresh a long time and in the past they were used for shipping meat and fruit before refrigerated containers were available.

Since ferns develop their leaves or rhythmic organs so much, one would expect them to have healing effects on rhythmic processes. However, they mostly work on metabolic rhythms, since the leaves retain processes that higher plants direct towards the formation of flowers.

In fact, herbalists in the Middle Ages often referred to the effect of various ferns on the spleen. According to Rudolf Steiner, the spleen is the organ that overcomes the foreign rhythms of ingested foods and brings them into the rhythms of the body.[4] Rudolf Steiner recommended a remedy that is prepared from the leaves of various ferns and willows to counteract disorder in digestive rhythms ranging from heartburn to constipation. Here male fern (Dryopteris Filix-mas) is assigned more to the stomach region and bracken more to the intestines. Ferns produce substances that have an inhibiting, shaping and consolidating effect upon digestive rhythms and others that accelerate, dissolve and dampen them. The first group includes tannins and the second essential oils. The stimulation of rhythmic processes results from the interaction between these two poles.

The digestive tract reflects the threefolding in man's overall body. The most conscious part of the digestive process takes place in the head and neck with its tasting, conscious chewing and swallowing movements. Man's I organization is active in the digestion of carbohydrates that begins in the mouth. The stomach is the central rhythmic organ and the "heart" of outer digestion, and it is not for nothing that it is located in the same region as man's main rhythmic organs, the heart and lungs, with its production of acids, the integration into the rhythm of waking and sleeping, its tasting process that is almost unconscious, etc.; it is an organ that is mainly taken hold by the astral body. Whereas the intestinal tract that is fully active even during sleep, with its processes that take place in

---

[4] See L. Kolisko, *Milzfunktion und Blutplättchenfrage*

complete unconsciousness, mainly reveals etheric activity. It also gives the completely liquefied and broken down food over to the enlivening process in the human etheric body.

According to Rudolf Steiner, the stronger, astralized male fern works more upon the stomach, and the bracken that is more devoted to etheric processes works upon the intestines. The interaction of the etheric and astral organizations that come to expression in the rhythmic activity of the digestive system is harmonized by fern preparations; it is accelerated if it is too slow and restrained if it is too fast. These preparations also counteract an overgrowth of microflora in the intestines. For ferns also push their own lower plant nature down below their higher one.

However, an equilibrium between anabolic etheric activity and catabolic astral activity must be maintained in each human organ in a different way for each. A predominance of proliferating plant processes leads to formlessness; a predominance of astral activity leads to excessive shaping, desiccation and devitalization. If the first occurs in a kidney, Rudolf Steiner recommended the use of a preparation from the very silica–rich bracken in order to tone down the excessive anabolic forces. In the opposite case one can use equisetum arvense, for by contrast with bracken it permeates its silica process with a powerful sulfur process. (See the section on medicinal plants for the kidneys below, where equisetum is described.)

The astral body is incorporated into man's body by three organs – through the nervous system as an entity that carries our consciousness, through the lung system as an entity that stimulates breathing, and through the kidney system as an entity that builds up the metabolic part of man. If the organs become impermeable for the working in of the astral body and astral activity is held up by these organs, it becomes physically manifest as cramps and psychologically manifest as soul abnormalities and disruptions of consciousness. Rudolf Steiner recommended a preparation of ferns and arum root for the treatment of such conditions, presumably for ones that were brought about by the kidneys.

Whereas we have so far only pointed to medications that are prepared from fern leaves and therefore from the highest, most perfect part of a fern through which it raises itself into the realm of the higher plants, Rudolf Steiner clearly composed a remedy for certain bone diseases (e.g. osteoporosis) where one uses fern spores or that part of the fern process that the leaf throws out, and out of which the lower animal-plant nature of ferns develops. The spores are worked up with fly agaric, oyster shells, silver and with potentized phosphorus (Agaricus comp./Phosphorus). The latter and the oyster shells have a connection with the bone building process and silver counteracts the inflammatory breakdown processes that accompany the bone diseases that were mentioned; we already mentioned that fungi can have a tissue regenerating effect. The lower plant side of ferns, the spores, probably work in the same direction. A bone is mainly an earth organ; only beings that live on the solid, mineral earth achieve a proper bone formation. This bone formation is undermined and reversed, as it were, in the disease referred to; the formative tendencies of an older phase of evolution assert themselves. They can be overcome through the activity of plants which themselves come from this older evolutionary stage of the earth and man.

HORSETAILS – EQUISETINAE

We will describe the horsetails in the section about curative plants for kidneys.

Medicinal Plants from the Upper Plant Kingdom

Evergreen Trees and Shrubs – Coniferae

A walk through an evergreen forest puts us into the primal mood of nature's existence, out of which a melody of long past days of creation ascends, weaving in the solemn blowing of the wind. Wonderful columns bear the tremendous vault of heaven, and a smell of incense wafts between the tree trunks. The many registers of a tremendous organ resound; when it stops a most reverent silence listens, and the wanderer's heart wants to bring a sacrifice to the altar as it is overcome by "the oldest, primal and most serious feelings of creation."[5]

It is really the case that when one goes through an evergreen forest one's soul is taken hold by feelings that are similar to the ones Goethe had when he stood on a granite peak and surveyed the sky above and the ground below. It seems to be as ancient as Saturn and like something that will last forever, and it is in fact resting on primal rock. A soul whose feelings have been shaken by the vicissitudes of life finds in it solitary quiet, forces that order its destiny and strengthen the I. Where can one find a more perfect vertical state? It is the one into which our I is always trying to place our bodies. That is why the old German store of words had the same word for firs and human beings: *Firaha*.[6]

A tremendous evergreen forest girdles the earth's northern temperate zone, and there is a somewhat smaller one in the southern temperate zone, due to the narrowness of the continents down there. The conifer areas in Alaska, Canada, Scandinavia, Russia and Siberia in the north are confronted by the ones in Chile, Tasmania and New Zealand in the south. The mountains' forests in the two temperate zones extend these girdles towards the south and north – just think of Italy's pines and cypresses, Greece's fir forests, Syria's pine forests, the cedars in Lebanon and on the Atlas mountains, Himalayan spruce, Japan's temple cypresses, Australia's sandarac cypress pines, California's giant trees, the spruce and pines in the Mexican mountains, the cypresses in Florida's swamps and the Araucarian pine forests on Brazil's mountains. Most of the conifers in the tropics are on high mountains. The scrub pines and junipers near the

---

[5] Goethe, *On Granite*
[6] Hegi, *Flora von Mitteleuropa*, Central European Flowers, Vol. 1, p. 597

timberline have their own kind of life, with their crowns pressed down to the rocky soil. They can do without upward–striving trunks because this tendency is more than compensated for by the towering rocks. But just transplant a dwarf pine into your front yard in the lowlands and it will grow into a little tree in a few years.

There is something sublime about the simplicity of coniferous trees. The greatest emphasis is placed upon the vertical wood formation in the trunk, and everything else is subordinate to that. The trunk is surrounded by branches that are like obliquely placed accessory trunks which circle around it like orbiting moons. The basic shape of the branching is strictly adhered to, and so the admirable multicrowns that extend in every direction in deciduous trees, are absent. The linear element predominates in them, and this enables one to cut the straightest and most elastic boards and beams from their trunks. This linear tendency only allows for the formation of needle–like or scaly leaves close to the twig, which are arranged in spirals around it and sometimes are hardly separated from it or are partially fused with it. One sometimes notices that they and the twig are contracted into green scales that make them look something like flat leaves, as one sees in Northern white cedar (Arbor vitae, Thuja occid.). The conifers include the tallest and oldest trees on earth, and even their needles can get to be up to 10 years old (Araucarian pines). Some giant sequoias are over 3000 years old, and their heights compete with those of the tallest church spires. The trunks of some species are practically indestructible, the wood in some Podocorpus trees that had been cut down and left in the forest decades ago in New Zealand was still completely usable, and in Silesia trunks of some extinct cypresses were salvaged from a lignite (wood Coal) lode, that could still be made into furniture.

The flowering process cannot change such a basic form very much; cones at the flowering stage look like things that are closely surrounded by lignified leaves and that have contracted into a cone or even a sphere that bears naked anthers or pistils which produce naked seeds for years. The whole class or subdivision of gymnosperms to which the conifer order belongs gets its name from the fact that it bears naked seeds.

Thus the woody principle presses up into flower formation, and the petals lignify. But what grew up so unswervingly surrenders to the upper elements; conifers are pollinated by the wind. A softening process produces fleshy scales in some species of needles and it can also affect the leaves or tissues that are close to the seed formations and produce juicy, berrylike fruits as in the case of yews and junipers. We become aware of a driving lignification process that produces soft wood.

In order to round out our understanding of conifers we will have to become aware of their close connection with the warmth element. The latter facilitates the formation of characteristic essential oils that permeate the needles and in some cases also the wood, cones or berries. Just think of the fragrant aromas from the oils in spruce needles, dwarf pines, juniper berries and cedar wood. This warmth process also calls forth resin formation in the branches, needles and trunks of conifers. Some species develop so much resin that it drips out of their cones. Turpentine, another etheric oil, can be obtained by cutting into balsam bark.

Those who have read my Healing Plants, Volume 1, will recall a number of descriptions of the unique plant process that expresses itself in the formation of essential oils, and they will also remember that a weaving of cosmic warmth into plant life and into the flower and fruit region is necessary for this formation. A plant's etheric or formative forces body directs its activities towards the earth and up towards the cosmos. It takes hold of the earthy and watery elements with life ether and chemical ether forces through root formation, working into the air and the cosmic light and warmth regions but with light ether and warmth ether. Thereby it develops the flower and fruit organs which collect cosmic forces in the same way that roots collect earthly forces. Germs and sprouts arise through the impulses from life and chemical ethers, leaves and their activities are indwelled by chemical and light ethers, and the formation of flowers and the ripening of fruits are induced by light and warmth ethers. Thus in primal plants one can have a harmonious interaction of the four formative forces of which their etheric bodies are composed, just as the physical body consists of solids, liquids, gases, etc. However, various manifestations of the archetypal plant can develop this or that process in a one–sided way and can let others atrophy; for instance, some families emphasize warmth processes and can therefore be called warmth plants. Labiates are an example of the latter, as we saw in Volume 1. The conifers can be added to this, and later we will see that the rues are a third warmth group. However, warmth works in these three large families in very different ways. Rues unite with tropical warmth process, labiates with those in the temperate zones, and conifers with those in cold climates – which seems to be a contradiction at first; but northern territories also have summers, with a great deal of light, where one can have midnight suns, and "white nights". The earth's highly differentiated warmth organizations confers its specialized warmth qualities to the plants at each particular place. This also becomes manifest in the various aromas characteristic of orange trees (rues), peppermints (labiates) and dwarf pines.

There is something special about an organism's capacity to draw cosmic warmth forces into its life processes in a cold climate to such an extent that it leads to the formation of large amounts of volatile oils and resins and to a kind of inner life fire that can defy long winters and great cold. This is where one can see the "saturnine" character of coniferous plants. The mighty Saturn which moves slowly, records everything and preserves a memory of an initial warmth stage of evolution. For more details about this see Rudolf Steiner's *Occult Science* in the chapter on cosmic and human evolution. Saturn preserves the sun's power of warmth at a great distance away from it, and it influences coniferous trees more than any other plant. The solemn feelings that one has upon seeing a cathedral of firs above and feeling connected with the primal depths of creation, are an inkling of the spiritual nature of the planetary power that is the godfather of the conifers.

The conifer's healing power is also based on the vital warmth processes that enter into the creation of ethereal oils and balsam resins. Briefly stated, they can promote the I's permeation of the warmth organization, and they have a warming, vitalizing effect. Here the plant being that prefers certain regions of the earth's warmth organization also looks for "its place" in our warmth organism with respect to its pharmacological effect. We find the body's cool region in the nervous system, which must nevertheless be vitalized and warmed through in the way that is appropriate for it. These are probably the effects that we mean when we speak of the nerve strengthening effect of a bath with spruce fir or dwarf pine extracts. Conifer oils can also be used to treat rheumatic ailments, hardening diseases and colds. We will go into more details about this when we discuss the most important healing plants in the family.

Something else that is connected with the inner warmth nature of conifer trees is the capacity to form fatty oils in the seeds, and to provide an important nut food: the European reader will be familiar with the cedar nuts from the Southern Alps and with Italy's pine nuts. The South American Araucaria bears head–sized cones with hundreds of large seeds which are a major source of food for some Indian tribes who even grind them into meal. Something similar could be said about Australian varieties.

*

Compared with other classes the coniferae class is not very large; it only has about 370 species. The type represents an important motif that is incapable of very much change. Usteri, the anthroposophic authority in botany, divides the main family into three genera.[7]

The Araucaria pines are the most primitive and primeval of these with 37 species which grow in the mountainous regions of Chile, Brazil, New Zealand, Australia and New Guinea. The reader is familiar with indoor firs with their regular, somewhat rigid growth, and he may have seen the stiff Araucarian pines from Chile in a botanical garden with the strange branches that are arranged like a candelabra. The famous, giant Agathis pines in New Zealand and the Philippines with their unusually wide needles produce Kauri gum or Manila copal that is similar to amber.

A second genus mentioned by Usteri are the Taxoceae or yews with 70 species. These conifers have no resin ducts in their needles and their cones do not lignify. They surround the carpel with a fleshy mantle like the ones on the red "berries" of our female yew trees. Species that look like ferns or club moss are among this archaic looking genus that lives mainly on the southern continents and in Eastern Asia. The formation of volatile oils and resins has been driven out of the leaves, although some species have resinous branches and some of the pseudo-berries taste like turpentine. However, this group has no medicinal value and so there is no point in discussing it further here.

The Pinaceae with 284 species is the largest group among the coniferous trees. The most important genera are the pines (70 species); spruces (26 species), firs (19 species), hemlocks (10 species), larches (12 species), cedar (2 species), the taxadioceae which includes Sequoia, Japanese and Taiwan cedars, and swamp cypress (3 species). Cypresses with opposite or whirled needles or fleshy scales exhibit a new possibility in this class, namely, succulent congestion. For instance, Thuja branches with their slimy, juicy, scaly leaves with much of their length attached to the twig are reminiscent of sedum or cactus-like formations. The young tree still has whole needles. Something similar appears to incense cedars,

---

[7] Usteri, *System der Phanerogamen*

cypresses and pseudo cypress. These conifer genera concentrate on trunk formation and produce especially solid wood. They do not dare to move out into hotter, drier parts of their growing places in the Mediterranean, Asia Minor, South Africa, Cape of Good Hope, India and California. The plastic power of the watery element has taken hold of leaf formation here. But this does not mean that their inner fiery force has been quenched; there are plenty of fragrant woods and no lack of resins and volatile oils. This softening, plastic force works on Juniper fruits, which have become fleshy, berrylike formations, and not just on their leaves. Junipers have needles, and creeping juniper has fleshy leaf scales that are something like the ones on Thuja. The long time it takes their "berries" to mature shows that they are really more like the wooden cones of the other conifers. We will now give a brief description of the therapeutically most important conifers.

The Pine family – Pinaceae

The subfamily of Abietineae includes spruce, fir, dwarf pines, and larches, which can be discussed together as medicinal plants since the most important thing about them is the formation of volatile oils and balsamic resins, and the weaving of cosmic warmth and light processes into these plants in the earth's cold zones. They all form a bit of Vitamin C, like all plants that have congestions, delays in biorhythms and in the formation of proteins, etc., due to unfavorable living conditions from which they cure themselves through the counter-action of energizing sulfur processes.

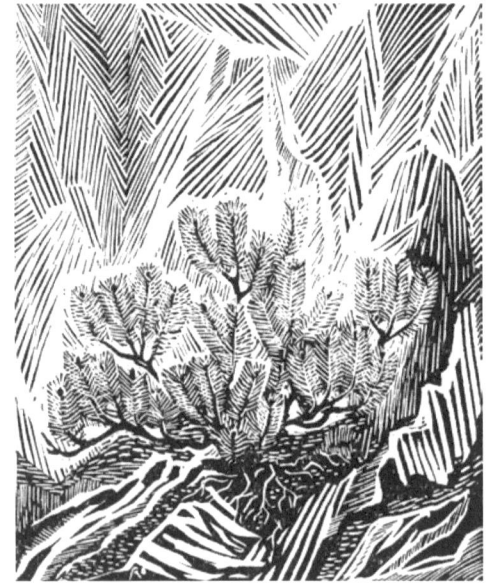

See the discussions about Vitamin C in Volume I of this work, especially in the chapter about Cruciferae, and also later on here in the section about Sea Buckthorn. What sulfur and sulfurous mustard oils do for Cruciferae, cosmic sulfur, warmth and light processes do for the Abietineae.

The essential oils that are obtained from the needles through steam distillation are the most important product from spruce, fir and dwarf pine, whereas balsamic larch resins are obtained by tapping the trunks.

What Rudolf Steiner once said about baths with the addition of fir needle extracts applies to the above essential oils in general, they stimulate the nervous system so much that it becomes somewhat emancipated and independent. That is what the previously mentioned nerve strengthening effect of the conifer's volatile oils is based on. Of course, it will make a slight difference as to whether one gets the oil from the needles of spruces which solemnly incline towards the earth and which like the moist and cool atmosphere, rather than from firs that strive defiantly upwards towards the light, or from the dwarf pines that climb up cliffs near the timber line. The latter have the strongest and yet finest aroma. That is why one often adds mixtures of these three oils to therapeutic baths.

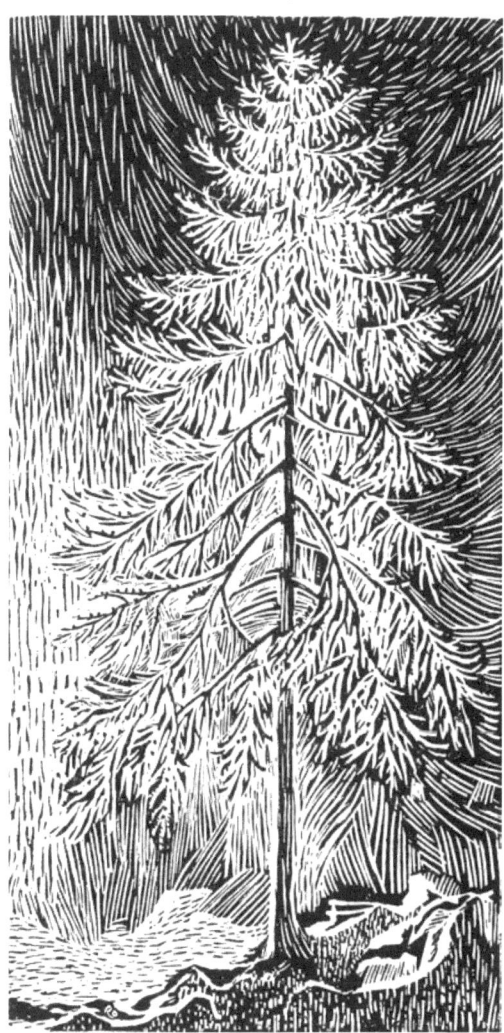

Rudolf Steiner recommended a fir resin

in the treatment of diabetes. It probably has an I-strengthening effect like that of rosemary, the "fir among labiatae".

Larches fall out of this series due to the shorter lifespan of their needles. They have adapted more to the sun's rhythm, and their needles only live for one year. They belong to weaving light more closely than the other Abietineae do; a grove of larches lets about as much light through as a birch forest does, and one would like to call the larch the birch among the evergreen trees. It strives for the sunny mountain tops in its growing places; it is a real mountain tree. It sends the forces of permanence, that it withholds from its leaves, all the more into the straight, high rising trunks that contain an almost imperishable wood that does not ever rot in water. Larches do not make much etheric oil in their leaves, but they produce plenty of balsamic resin obtained by tapping their trunks. From this resin one can then extract "Venetian turpentine."

Rudolf Steiner once said something fundamental about the three kinds of sap that course through trees in a lecture to the workmen at the Goetheanum.[8] The earth life presses into the tree through the roots together with ground water and specifically chosen ground salts that are dissolved into an earth sap, which dies in the wood and trunk formation. (The earth is not looked upon as a dead clump of minerals here, but as a gigantic living being that has a formative forces body in addition to the physical body that people usually focus on to the exclusion of the first one. (See the books by G. Wachsmuth, W. Cloos, etc. that are often mentioned for this.)   Now while the dissolved solids in the earth sap rise in the plant, lose their life and turn into wood, a life sap forms through the leaves' activity in the weaving together of fluids and air, which circles around the vertical trunk, as one can see from the way the leaves are arranged.   While the earth sap or wood sap streams up and dies in the formation of the trunk, the plant becomes re–enlivened through the spiraling process of the life–sap formation.

The latter process stimulates an inner warmth process that becomes a formation of resin and plant gum that unites with the formation of a third sap in the cambium. Whereas the earth sap is connected with the earth's forces and the life–sap is connected with the surrounding atmospheric forces, the sap in the cambium connects the plant with the starry environment and therefore with the spiritual formative forces of the particular

---

[8] *Cosmic Workings in Earth and Man.* Lecture 5

plant, which can then be conveyed to the seed formation. Elsewhere in this book one will see how the cosmic warmth in the hydrogen process finds an earthy carrier substance, and one can say that the seed formation process is a hydrogen process that has been elevated to the stage of plant life. On the other hand the formation of essential oils that is combined with resin formation is also a warmth and hydrogen process.

When one taps into the larch's cambium layer between its wood and bark, and obtains its balsam sap, one has an imprint of all the stars' formative forces in it, with which the larch's spiritual formative principle has sunk into the plant's body via the warmth. Larches have a more intensive silica process than the other coniferous trees, although one finds a fair amount of silica in the ashes of all of them. Larches have the light, and let more light through their branches than other conifers do. This gives a special quality to larch resin, and it enables one to see why Rudolf Steiner recommended larch resin as a remedy for the sensory sphere. (Larch resin, pineapple juice and lavender oil, or a combination of larch resin and wormwood for the treatment of inflamed eye lids; larch resin, elderberry pith and lilac blossoms (*Syringa vulgaris*) for psoriasis, etc.)

Cypress-like Shrubs and Trees – Cypressaceae

We will mention two genera of this subfamily of Coniferales for its healing potential, Thuja and junipers.

Thuja occidentalis – Northern White Cedar (Arbor Vitae)

The needle formation in the twigs is held back by the tough life forces with which this moderately tall tree is filled. The young plants still have short, juniper-like needles, but then the leaf anlage turns into fleshy scales, and the terminal twigs take on a leafy appearance, like pinnate fern leaves; they spread out into horizontal surfaces (whereas Thuja orientalis puts out vertical leaf twig surfaces.) This coniferous tree is taken hold by the succulent principle, it shows a congestion in the watery element. This also becomes manifest in a mighty formation of glycides; the needle juice is full of mucilage. Our plant's strong vital force also makes it into a luxuriantly sprouting hedge bush that forms dense, green walls.

The flowers and woody cones with only a few scales are quite small. The cosmic warmth element finds it harder to work its way into plants with watery, mucilagenous congestion than into typical conifers. The essential oils which form are coarser, stronger and more aromatic than in spruce, fir and pine. They have something inflammatory about them. So this process of volatile oil formation did in fact succeed in penetrating into the region of life congestion and mucilage formation.

Thuja can work upon the kind of human processes in which there is a major interaction between the I organization and the life body or etheric body. The volatile oils that are born from warmth stimulate the I organization which lives in the warmth configuration of the human body. Thuja is good for certain forms of digestive weakness. According to an indication by Rudolf Steiner, Thuja can be a considerable help in cases where foods are not tasted intensively enough, so that they are not broken down sufficiently during digestion or dissolved in digestive juices enough or divested of their own life enough. Therefore they cannot be taken hold of enough by man's etheric body, and cannot make a proper transition from the digestive system into the inner formation of lymph and blood. Of course an appropriate pharmaceutical elaboration and a small dose is necessary, otherwise Thuja can produce severe inflammations in the lower organs that might even be fatal, with damage to the liver, in which warmth and liquid processes and the I and astral body interact in a particularly intensive way.

Juniperus communis – Dwarf Juniper

Dwarf Juniper is a tree, or more commonly a shrub, on German heaths and moors, rocky mountain meadows and slopes in the Jura Mountains, as well as in similar landscapes in other northern continents. The small tree or shrub bears its lively vitality with a serious dignity and ceremoniousness on fertile soils and covers them with bushy groves and thorny preserves. But it is just as aromatic as its taller relatives. Its wood and berries furnish a strong incense and a spice that help one to digest cabbage, Sauerkraut and other flatulent foods. Rudolf Steiner recommended baths containing a decoction of juniper berries, fir needles and elderberry blossoms for sensitive nerves, and injections of preparations of juniper berries and sloes.

In past times people who felt that the forces of nature in desolate, infertile landscapes were demonic looked upon our dwarf among the conifers as something good, that awakened vital forces, had a warming and powerful form and that cleared the way for friendly beings in Nature. Its aroma and appearance were enough to strengthen one's consciousness and to drive away spooks. The "tree singer" in the old Christmas plays led his actors onto the stage carrying a little juniper bush that was decorated with ribbons. This stage represented the paradisical world in which the creation, temptation and fall into sin of Adam and Eve took place. The best thing stood in the middle of the garden in Paradise which contained all the trees, it was the Tree of Knowledge with its enticing fruits and the Tempter in it branches..However, the juniper bush in the tree singer's hand was like a salutary counter image, a foreshadowing of the coming of our Christmas tree,

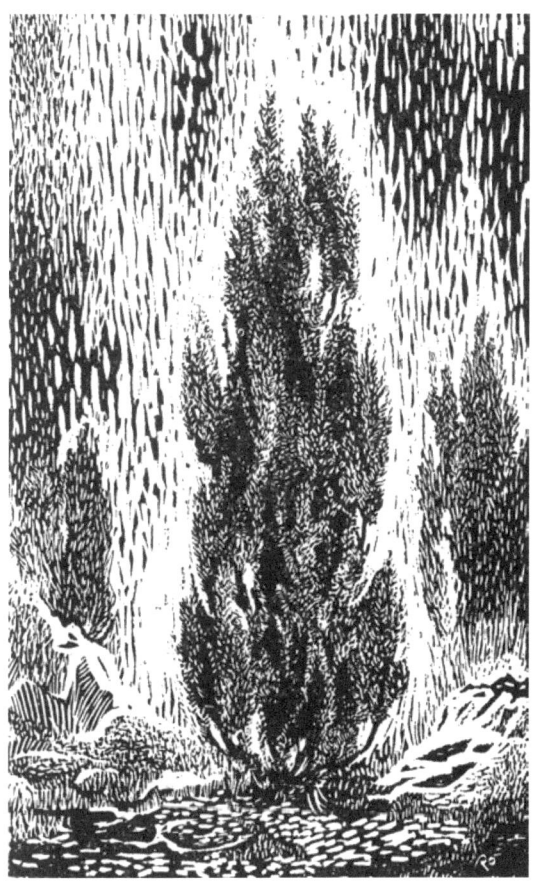

under which we place a crib with the images of a new Paradise seed, a human couple from whom we were given the fruit that overcomes the fall into sin. Animals assembled peacefully and plants grow around the crib, and the tree of life protects them. The tree singer carries a juniper as an image of the Paradise and the life tree that can be attained again in the future through Christ. The juniper pricks one like a crown of thorns and its tart, berrylike and inconspicuous fruits are concealed in scaly leaves, but they are bitter and salutary if we have become sick to our stomachs with the sweet, sensory feasts of the earth.

Juniperus Sabina – *Creeping Juniper*

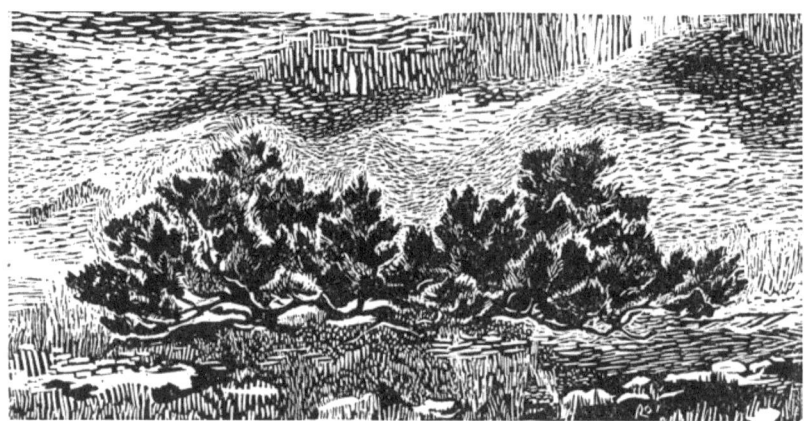

Conifers are divided into the Pine type and the Cypress type with regard to their typical growth forms. The latter kind emphasizes the vertical element or the sun line of straight trunks, whereas the former has a horizontal umbrella and a "planetary principle" for its encircling branches. Juniper manikins look like cypresses, whereas the very ramified, creeping juniper, the "baby killer," imitates the pines' gesture. Although its ripe bluish blackberries show that it is a juniper, it is quite a contrast to juniper communis. Its scaly leaves are pressed close to the twigs and look something like Thuja species. In spite of the hint of a cedar fragrance, its aroma is pungent, repulsive and mildly stimulating. The volatile oil and even the decoction from the leaves have a corrosive, inflammatory effect, and if taken internally, produce blood congestion in the abdominal organs and severe inflammatory symptoms with intestinal, kidney and uterine bleeding that can lead to miscarriages and to the mother's death. Creeping juniper shows that conifers can become poisonous plants. It is a "juniper that has become insidious." The conifer being distinguishes itself through the formation of volatile oils (which are otherwise characteristic for the flowering process) right into the leaves and wood. It cannot yet develop the flowers of higher plants, but thanks to its connections with light and warmth it already has the fiery quality of blossoms in its stem and leaves, and that is why it has such a stimulating effect on our warmth organism. This is intensified to a toxic effect in Juniperus sabina.

*

St. John's Worts – Guttiferae

The typical aspect of St. John's worts is their strong flowering nature that is not just active as an upper nature in numerous, large blossomed, bright colored, often fragrant inflorescence, but it is also active in a different way in the resin, balsam and yellow sap in the leaves, stems, trunks, bark and roots and it thereby sinks way down into their lower nature. However, there is considerable condensation and solidification in their lower nature; one can find numerous high rising trees with wood as hard as iron among the 800 plus species in this family; even the St. John's worts in Germany and the Mediterranean countries have tough, hard stems, which is reflected in their common name Harthen, hard hay.

So what one sees is something that is rigidified into fluids and solids, and it is not a flaring up and dying down of things that have been created by warmth and light. The fluidic element is tightly pulled together here, and it does not flow in a sumptuous and plastic way. It is permeated by light and fragrances, volatile oils and orange gum resins appear.

The family is mainly tropical in distribution in places where the earth draws in cosmic elements intensively and pushes itself up into them and thereby makes them earthy. That is where the Guttiferae trees and shrubs are. In the temperate zones they are subshrubs or herbs which bloom around St. John's tide.

Guttiferae leaves are simple, undivided, often leathery and sometimes contracted into needle. The separate petals of the flowers are large, yellow, white or rose colored; they are located at the ends of radially symmetrical branches, mostly in panicles. But the unique thing about the Guttiferae is the large number of formative forces in their anther or stamen region. This simple, linear organ is not only produced in large numbers in them – it is used as material for formations in which the species of this family disclose their nature. The forest of anthers is divided into groups and they are physically shaped into tubes, cups, hemispheres, columns, collars, spheres, clubs, bottles and cones, – what otherwise comes to expression in the three dimensional plasticity of flowers and even more in the fruit takes hold of the antheral realm here. The stigmas participate in this process to a lesser extent and some of them look like heads, clubs, funnels and lobed shields or caps. The Guttiferae show their capacity for shaping themselves in their anthers just as the orchids indicate this in their flowers, ferns in their leaves and Cruciferae in their fruit forms. One sees here formative forces in the volatilization realm where plant pollen passes over into an airy element that is permeated with astrality. The Guttiferae do a lot of intensive shaping in this area.

Most of their fruits are dry capsules, but some species have juicy, acidic, aromatic fruits. Mangosteen shrubs bear one of the best tasting tropical fruits. The tasty seed mantle or flesh covers oily seeds under a thick rind that is full of guttifer juice. The family in general has a lot of oily seeds, a strong elaboration of warmth is expressed in this; the suet trees in East and West Africa are good examples. The bitter aromatic seeds of Garcinia Cola or bitter cola are full of resin ducts; this cola nut is highly valued by the natives of Central Africa as a stimulant. Maria balsam and other balsams that flow out of cuts in tropical tree trunks are often used as external remedies for wounds, and saps that contain resins and gum resins (gamboge) are used internally as an antihelminthic. We will only give a more detailed description here of the essential nature of St. John's wort. That famous healing and wound herb which we now know a little more about through the medicine that has been extended by spiritual science.

Hypericum perforatum – The genuine St. John's Wort

One thing that is certain is that the noble medicinal plant under discussion here belongs to the light side of earth life. The seeds can only germinate in bright light, and in dark places they can lie in moist earth for years without doing anything. It likes light filled, dry, barren soil, the edge of woods and paths, banks, illumined bushes, clearings, moss covered piles of rocks and the like. The root of the plant with a perennial rhizome dives powerfully down into the ground; the shoot that comes up in the spring is erect with an umbrella of branches higher up, so that it looks something like an inverted pyramid, it gets broader up there and is crowned with numerous golden yellow flowers that are arranged in panicles. The leaves are little, pointed, elliptical formations without stipules and with blackish glands at their edges; when held up to the light they are dotted with transparent oil glands and at first glance they seem to be perforated. The sepals are also dotted with light and dark glands, the flower stalks are black with glands, even the sunny yellow petals are covered with fine, dark points and streaks – oil glands all – especially on the wider, bulging side. The five petals are not symmetrically formed. They have a sharper half and a widely outstretched half – something like plane propellers – which makes the flower look like a pinwheel or a sun gear, as if it were going to start revolving slowly at any moment.

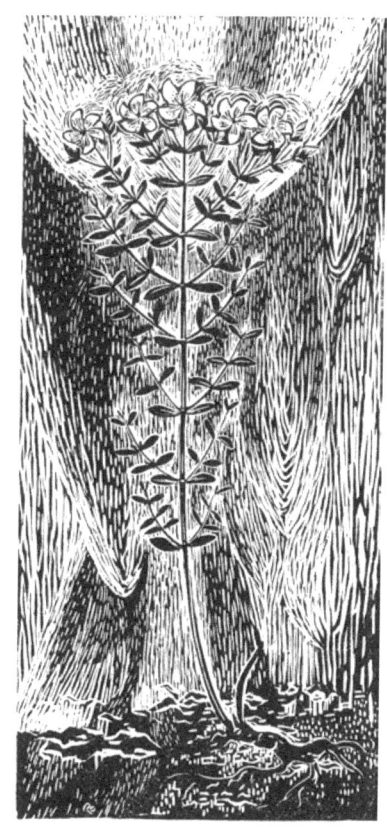

Such a rotation actually occurs when the flower opens, since the petals are folded into the bud in a spiral way. The numerous stamens are arranged in three bundles, the so–called ovary has a tripartite stigma. The heart–shaped, pointed capsule contains light, blackish seeds about 1 mm in diameter. Everything in the upper part of this plant passes over into levity and light. The opening flower announces St. John's tide, the high point of the year. The full strength of the summer sun lives in it. One can recognize this plant at quite a distance through this sunny radiance and also through its slender, erect growth, its rigid, solid and tough stem, and its well–formed and magnificently ordered appearance. All of this makes it into one of the most beautiful midsummer plants.

In the fall its vitality sinks into its lower organs and while the part above ground dies the rhizome sends out new shoots with leaves on the ground that survive the winter. Thus, like Arnica, the organs that belong to the root region are particularly vigorous.

St. John's wort used to be treasured highly and Paracelsus sang its praises. It was known how to interpret the language of the forces weaving in it through its whole appearance and its "sensory, moral impression." This was forgotten by a later generation that only accepted what can be placed upon a scale: even though people still gathered its flowers and placed them in sunlight with oil in order to obtain the red oil that helps to heal wounds, burns, cramps and nerve pains. People started to take it seriously again when chemists found a number of tannins, bitter substances, and some volatile oil in the bright glands that make the leaves look like they have been pierced. It also contains resinous materials and the dark glands contain the bright red, fluorescent dye, hypericin. The latter has the peculiar property that whereas animals who eat small amounts of it are not adversely affected as long as they stay in dark places, as soon as they go into the light they get cramps and eventually die. Animals with white spots on their skin or hair who eat too much St. John's wort out on the fields can get inflammatory swellings on these white places. Black sheep may survive but white ones die; thus light becomes a poison for them through the hypericin. The peripheral skin process that otherwise stops the effect of outer light is penetrated, and light becomes transformed and "digested". The organism is thereby overpowered by the outer light, which goes into the skin like a foreign body, and the organism defends itself against it through an inflammation and through a strengthening of its blood process, as it would against any foreign body. In the formation of hypericin one becomes aware of the special relation that Hypericum perforatum has to the annual, cosmic light processes. It surrenders itself to them almost too much, but it also weakens them and banishes the excess light into the red dyes that are secreted into the glands that look black.

Rudolf Steiner compared the healing effect of the bitter substance that is extracted from the flowering Hypericum and suitably prepared with that of arsenic, one of the strongest mineral remedies. He said that arsenic energized the astral body. It stimulates considerable movement in it, albeit for a short time. However if it is used more carefully, arsenic can promote digestion, stimulate blood formation and strengthen one's consciousness. Through its material properties arsenic enables the astral body to move into the physical body, and to take hold of it more intensively. As we mentioned in the introductory sections of Volume I of *Healing Plants*, the astral body incarnates in man's air organization and takes hold of the fluids and solids in him to the extent that they are connected with the airy element. Now arsenic is a semi-metallic substance that volatilizes very easily, without first melting, into a sulfurous vapor that smells like garlic; thus it suppresses the fluidic state and greedily enters the gaseous state. When it combines with other metals it eliminates their inner fluidity, plasticity and malleability and makes them hard and brittle. Thereby it supports the astral body's attempts to make etheric processes subordinate to it, to dampen flowing life, and to press form processes upon it which make the soul element, that controls life, become manifest in structures of the body. In a way one could call the astralizing activity an "arsenification". The process that once dampened the fluidically enlivened forms in the earth's life to such an extent that the latter excreted minerals and rocks with their rigid forms, was a cosmic arsenification, that went parallel with a greater permeation of the entire earth's life with astrality and with the development of higher animal forms, etc. (see R. Steiner's, *Spiritual Science and Medicine*, and the chapter on Cosmic and Human Evolution in *Occult Science*.)

Now the bitter substance that is extracted from St. John's Wort is similar to arsenic in that it works upon the astral body's inner mobility, but the effect lasts much longer. Among other things one can use it to treat bedwetters, that is, children who may tend to remain in the more unconscious, vital plant state of an infant and who have no control over their bladder functions. In addition there is the effect of the volatile oil upon our warmth and I organization and of the yellow carotine dye that carries the anabolic and digestive processes right into the realm of formative processes in the nerves and senses. Rudolf Steiner indicated the use of "primary yellow flowers" in the combating of malnutrition in the organs of the rhythmic system, and among these he mentioned primula veris (see below), bird's foot trefoil, and St. John's Wort. In connection with a discussion of arnica and calendula, he noted that carotene and the Vitamin A that comes from this, help to carry anabolic processes into the sphere of the nerves and senses, or into the silica region.

All of this makes Hypericum into a remedy for many nervous disorders such as shock to the brain and spinal cord, and for inadequate nutrition of nerves. It also contributes to wound healing and has proven its value for burns. Furthermore it is used as an agent for bringing the astral body into the sexual region so as to counteract menstrual disorders, menopausal problems, etc.

Three decades after Rudolf Steiner gave his indications, J. Klosa, reported in a medical journal that St. John's Wort "is a remedy that it would be difficult to replace with other medications, and its comprehensive value should gain more recognition. The results with hypericine can be compared with iron–arsenic therapy. However Hypericum as a phyto–psychotonicum (energizes the psyche or astral body) has the additional advantage of relative harmlessness." (*Die Heilkunst*, vol. 4, 1951). Thus a physician who observes things exactly arrives at the same description of hypericum's effect, the comparison with arsenic and an improved tone for the psyche that had been found and presented decades earlier through the methods of modern spiritual investigation.

As we have had to do so often before, we must expand our concepts here in order to understand the world processes that create substances and precede and bring about all material existence in the life of plants. This is not as obvious in the inorganic realm since most of the processes that created substances there have ceased. One has to speak of arsenic but also of the arsenic process, and with this concept one can characterize all events in which essential astral forces, that use aeriform things, penetrate the etheric activities that stream through fluids in such a way that they drive them into rigidification, solidification and hardening. As luxuriant as St. John's Worts are in their flowers, spraying anthers, aromas and colors, they are rather scraggly, taut and hard in their processes, and they are iron hard in their wood formation. What is between the blossom and trunk or stem has a tendency to contract and dry out. This can be called arsenification and the mineral arsenic gives a particularly clear demonstration of the arsenic process that has become inactive in the lifeless mineral realm.

Rock foil plants – Saxifragaceae

Silica process, limestone and light processes

A mountain climber gets a strange feeling when he encounters rockfoil species up in the heights; it is as if the cool, clear crystals that are concealed in the rocks had acquired the power to blossom and were displaying themselves in the magnificent, strict forms and the bright rays of color, as a starry world that was enchanted into the solid ground. Each rockfoil belongs to a particular kind of rock and therefore has a fairly narrowly circumscribed sphere of existence. Some grow on limestone, schist or granite, some on the highest ridges and cliffs and others in chasms, clefts and crevices. Some creep along ledges and others live on rocky debris or wet gravel. Some species wander down into the depths with the water falls, avalanches and sliding rocks and take root on rocky banks or fallen, mossy boulders. It is as if the power that breaks off rocks had called forth one species of rockfoil at every step of their activities as a testimonial to their deed, and to reinforce what they achieved, and as if every stage of the disintegration had liberated forces that could disclose something of their nature through such beautiful plants. Since the broken, weathered rock eventually becomes earth and mixes with plants to form humus, the saxifrage type also sends certain species down into the mountain meadows and woods, allows a few bushes to arise, and even grows some nice, leathery-leafed trees in our antipodes. But even here damp ravines and rocks are the favorite growing places. Most of the 800 plus species are mountain plants, especially in the main saxifrage genus with 300 species, which grow everywhere except past $83°$ north and south and above 20,000 feet in the Asian mountains. The genus Escallonia (45 species) in the Andes replaces Europe's Alpine roses.

Thus the elements that our type needs are light, rocks, water and low temperatures. It develops its tremendously vital lower organs towards the moist rocks and it has leaves that are contracted into rosettes, needles or scales on short petioles; these are formations that can combine into cushions, send out runners and thus vegetate further, and they can conjure up live oases in dead, rocky wastes. Torn off rosettes that get blown away can put down roots again elsewhere, and some species form breeding buds that can separate and form new plants. Thus the biological processes push down into the compressed lower organs and thereby maintain a certain amount of vitality. Here the minerals in the rocky soil can be attacked aggressively, dissolved in sap, and thereby raised to the life stage.

They can then be secreted towards the periphery through special glands, where white calcium carbonate crusts or fine dust becomes visible on the surfaces of the leaves.

The slender flower stems rise straight up from such congested lower organs, rosettes and cushions, which leave everything that cannot become a flower behind them down below and ray out clear, star forms in flowers that have the color of stars in the cosmic light. A hiker can really be moved by their chaste coolness and rejoice in their light. Their tiny seeds get scattered into the almost weightless air.

Once you get the feel for the type as a whole you will be able to feel your way into the variations, and be able to grasp

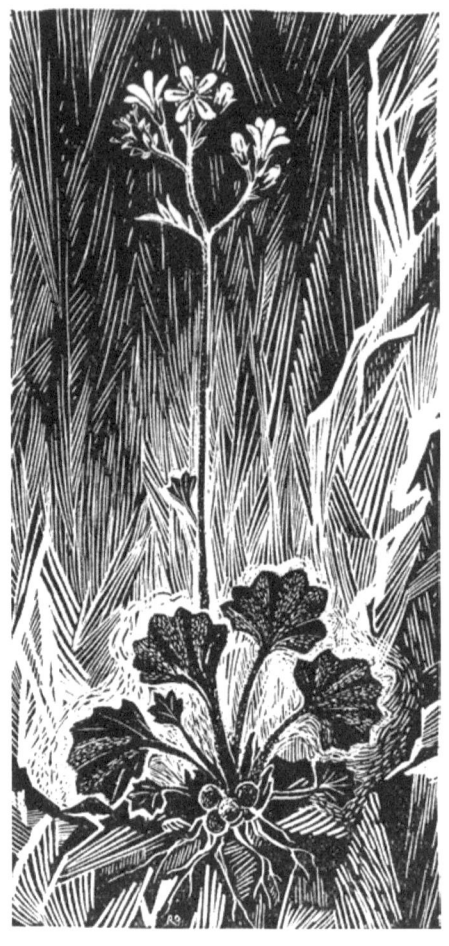

"saxifragedness" of the spleen herbs (chrysosplenium, 55 species). They are still quite close to the coldness of the winter and its cosmic forces (since they mainly grow in lower landscapes in the spring), but raise their golden-green leaf rosettes into the flower region and fuse them into a flowery unit with the little, yellow blossoms that form a calyx but not a corolla. Hortensia, a hydrangia species that is like a long spleen herb with much more luxuriant and colorful flowers, grows in the forests of southeast Asia and in North America. The type forms the pipe shrub varieties with their milky white, very fragrant flowers (Philadelphus, false jasmine) which still like rocky mountain forests and ravines. In gooseberries and currant bushes the saxifrageal rosette on the ground has become a bundle of short shoots which release a cluster of blossoms. In them the type becomes a giver of fruit, and it thereby shows its relation to rose plants. The fine airy flower clusters of the Astilbes that grow along mountain streams and the wet edges of forests look very similar to the Spireas among the Rosaceae.

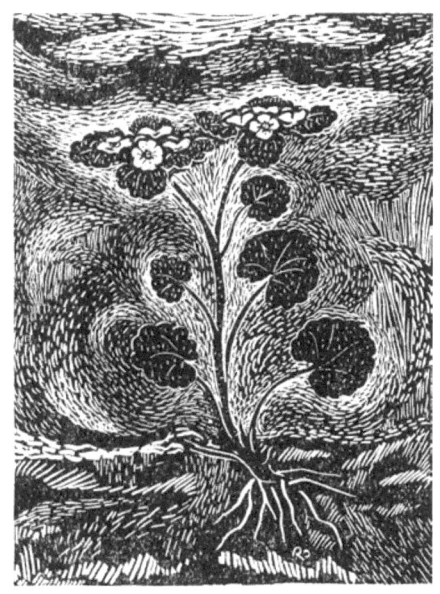

The Saxifragale being shows that a plant type that interacts with hard rocks to a great extent can also take in earthy solidification forces, through the fact that it produces a number of tree species. Some think that Tawapi trees (Ixerba brexioides) are the most beautiful ones in New Zealand. They are solid, strong and up to 50 feet high. The leathery, evergreen, long, narrow leaves, that are somewhat similar to chestnut leaves, gather round the ends of the twigs like rosettes and conceal the milky white, beautiful flowers with spraying anthers, that are grouped together like umbels; one recognizes saxifrage and spleen herbs in the metamorphosis. Meadow saxifrage and chrysosplenium were once used medicinally.

*

Thus rockfoil plants interact with the mineral rocks in an intensive way, especially with two fundamental processes that work through these rocks in the earth and which are a primary polarity in them. These are the silica and limestone processes or the siliceous and calciferous ones. These polarities are harmoniously connected in granite; the more acid a rock is the more the siliceous element predominates, and the more alkaline it is the more the calciferous element predominates. All plants are affected by these polarities, but this is especially obvious in rockfoils. The plants that grow on silica and limestone are quite different, as those who have read Volume I of this work will know quite well.

We run into silica and limestone substances in the dead mineral world. But these become living processes in the plants that take in these two substances; specific activities become connected with them and they "become raised to the stage of life". Rudolf Steiner gave us some particularly poignant descriptions of these fundamental processes that are so important for plant life. According to him the silica in the soil mediates cosmic effects to the plant and limestone mediates terrestrial effects. A plant is a mediating being between the cosmos and the earth. The heavenly world belongs to it being just as much as the earthly one does. Silica and limestone are two mighty helpers for it so that it can develop the two sides of its nature in a bodily, material form. Plants would have to have entirely different forms if there was less silica in the earth and its silica process was weaker, in which case they might look something like cactuses but with inconspicuous flowers. Growth would be confined to earthy stumps and it would not be able to receive the cosmic impulses that lead to the formation of flowers. The formation of food stuffs in particular would cease. However, if the earth did not develop enough limestone processes the terrestrial element would not enter the plants enough, and the right trunk formation would not occur (a trunk is "protruding earth"). Winding growths or vines would arise, which no doubt would have flowers, but their ability to reproduce would be low. The cosmic impulse for movement that is reflected in the spiral attachment of leaves to their shoots would take hold of the stems and trunks and would turn them into vines. A plant would devote itself to its cosmic archetype in its blossoms, but it would be unable to bring it down to earth in its ovaries, in the formation of many seeds.

The rockfoils indicate that they let silica and limestone work through them in a harmonious way. They have no inclination towards succulent congestion (as the related crassulaceae do) and they radiate an intensive flowering process; thus they use the silica process a great deal. Their "sense" is completely open for their cosmic environment. That is why they like high mountains and the far north. Their ability to create nutrients makes some of them into fruit. At the same time they are quite involved in the limestone process; they can draw in and enliven limestone and secrete it into their own calcium glands. They have strong reproductive forces in their seeds, runners, germinal buds and nodules.

The healing potential of the rockfoils results from such characteristics. Human nature needs more than enlivening, anabolic processes, for the latter would only enable us to vegetate. In order to develop consciousness and self–consciousness it must be able to tear down and devitalize life and to lead it over into death processes. Thereby the enlivened substances fall back down to the stage of lifeless minerals. These must be secreted from the organism. Hardening and the formation of stones should not occur in organisms. The inner cosmic nature of the human body should not let earthly forces penetrate it too much. It must produce the right relation of limestone processes to silica processes. If this is upset, as we can see in the formation of kidney stones, one can use rockfoils as remedies, as was done in the Middle Ages.

However, if one is a student of Nature and one takes its examinations, as it were, one can make something that is more effective if one adjusts the ratio of silica and limestone through a pharmaceutical process, and thereby calls forth a counter-process to the pathological formation of kidney stones. Rudolf Steiner indicated how such a remedy can be prepared. (Lapis cancri and flint mixture)

THICK-LEAFED PLANTS – CRASSULACEAE

The Succulence Phenomenon (watery congestion)
The Archetypal Plant and its Reflection in Bryophyllum

The phenomenon of the congestion of plant formation in the watery element and the exuberant swelling of surging life is not restricted to succulent plants, it is a process that practically every plant goes through in certain stages of its development, but it has been adhered to in Bryophyllum until it has become excessive. It first occurs at the germination stage when the seed that has been entrusted to the dark, damp ground soaks up the watery element, takes hold of and permeates it with its formative forces and becomes a spherically expanding drop of life, a swelling biohydrosphere. The cotyledons and hypocotyl are often thick, swollen and unformed. However, this condition rapidly changes in most plants. The drop becomes planar and turns into a proper, green leaf; the watery and airy elements touch each other in a plane. Thereby light and air are woven into the fluids, and formative forces are woven into formlessly welling life. Then the plant contracts into a flower and the cosmic sphere weaves its ripening powers into the "ovaries", where the plant swells up succulently for the second time, in the juicy fruit. (This stage is adhered to in berries but it is abandoned quickly in dry fruit.)

A struggle between the upper and lower formative forces always takes place in plants. The former work in light and air, the latter in the watery element. There has to be a transition from the hydrosphere into a formation of planes in order to open it up to air and light forces. Succulent plants do not make this transition, whereas the nonsucculent ones can make it in a harmonious way. The material drive (in Schiller's sense) accompanies the former event and the form drive accompanies the latter one. Succulent plants do not do justice to the form drive. That is why thick leafed plants are interesting but never very beautiful. The more succulent they are the more monstrous they are. We feel that a special cactus, a candelabric wolf's milk, a Stapelia or an Aloe are really misshapen; we are relieved at the gradual decongestion in the sedum species, but in spite of the gay colors and forms we can only say that they have a plump beauty and a stiff, crude magnificence.

The over 500 species of Crassulaceae retain the succulence stage of the germinal organs in all of their leaves. Their leaf formation process often congests and creates a rosette on the ground, and sometimes the latter pulls together into a spherical bud like a cabbage, as in house leek (sempervivum tectorum). A shooting up follows congesting sooner or later depending on the extent to which the congestion is retained. The flower bud ascends and divides inwardly into spikes or panicles, and finally bursts into bloom. The powerful flowering process announces – with white, yellow, yellowish red and red tones – that the sun's forces have been victorious over the lunar nature of the watery element after all the obstructions and delay. Now dry capsules form as fruit, and the wind scatters the tiny seeds.

The strong plastic vitality of this plant family does not permit any hardening and lignification; this type is incapable of forming trees, bushes or thorns. It also forms no parasitic plants; its own life forces are so strong and exuberant that it does not have to borrow anything from foreign life. On the contrary, it grow on desolate stones sterile, sandy soil, and bare rock all the way up into the mountains. The dry landscapes of South Africa produce an especially large number of Crassulaceae that like a lot of light and a hot sun. The strong vitality which comes to expression in the succulence easily repels the intervention of the "upper" cosmic sphere. The moist coolness does not permit combustible substances to form; we find no aromatic oils, balsams or resins in them. Due to the good "etheric cushioning" one does not get an excessive intervention of astral forces through the fairly intensive flowering process, and that is why Crassulaceae do not develop any poisons.

Crassulaceae bloom in the summer; the intensity of vernal, cosmic forces isn't great enough to make their congested organs shoot up. The cool beauties wait and then surrender themselves to the onslaught of the summer heat. The flowers retain some of the vitality of the leaves below them; they live quite a long time and wilt slowly.

The succulent's congestion in form is accompanied by a metabolic congestion that leads to the formation of particular plant acids. The oxygen respiration that runs parallel to the life process in every plant and which normally oxidizes the carbon in plants into carbon dioxide, stops in succulents at the last stage; and so in connection with the etheric congestion one gets a liberal formation of plant acids, especially of a certain kind of apple acid which is called Crassulaceamalic acid. (Fruit acids are also present in cacti, apples, berries, grapes and other succulent fruits.) Such acids are formed in Crassulaceae mainly at night. During the day they are converted to carbonic acid under the influence of the sun's light and warmth, and exhaled. The acids are also present in sour fruits in general, and as the sun ripens them the former are exhaled and the fruit becomes sweet. The formation of oxalic, citric, malic, ascorbic, succinic and other plant acids is always connected with the appearance of biological congestion and its elimination. In the first volume of this work we described the basic elements in proteins as substances for the incarnation of the plant's higher members. There we explained how oxygen facilitates the entry of etheric life forces into the physical world, and that this is why oxygen is so essential for all biological processes.

Since the forces that shape life become congested in succulence, one does not have too many metamorphoses in this plant family. Their leaves remain at the primitive stage of cotyledon, and the archetypal plant does not become manifest in transformations. However, the strong life forces of the germinal stage are retained, and they can move through the whole plant; this can be seen best in species of Bryophyllum, whose leaves can sprout new plants in the notches around their border, and they thereby show a thoughtful observer that the whole plant is present in every part of the plant's body. It is easy to see why the idea of the archetypal plant awakened in Goethe when he looked at this plant.

Bryophyllum calycinum – *Sprouting leaf plant*

This plant – and three other relatives in the small genus Bryophyllum – requires one to encounter it with reverence. After all Goethe's perception of it enabled him to intuit a fundamental law of all life, namely, that the wh ole is present and active in every part of an organism, or that the super spatial, super temporal, spiritual principle of the archetypal plant is active in each of its spatial, temporal manifestations. The etheric formative forces of this thick leafed herb that are congested in its succulence permit many little plants with roots to develop from the notches in the pointed ovoid leaves, which then fall off, become rooted and thus assure a plentiful supply of this tropical weed. The reproductive power that other "normal" plants withdraw from their leaves and concentrate on the place where flowers and fruit form, is poured over the entire plant. Just as a large drop of water disperses into many small ones, so the main plant scatters into many new ones at rhythmic intervals that are conditioned by the seasons. Nevertheless, the growth of the sprouting leaves is topped off by a well–developed cluster of many hanging reddish–yellow tubular flowers. They have practically no fragrance and are enclosed by long calyces. As in other thick–leafed plants, the strong congested etheric body is no hindrance to a well developed flowering process – the astral can still work into the sphere of the formative forces. However, growth must be supported by a lot of light and warmth such as one finds in climates where the tropical weed comes from, for it "freezes" at tempera-

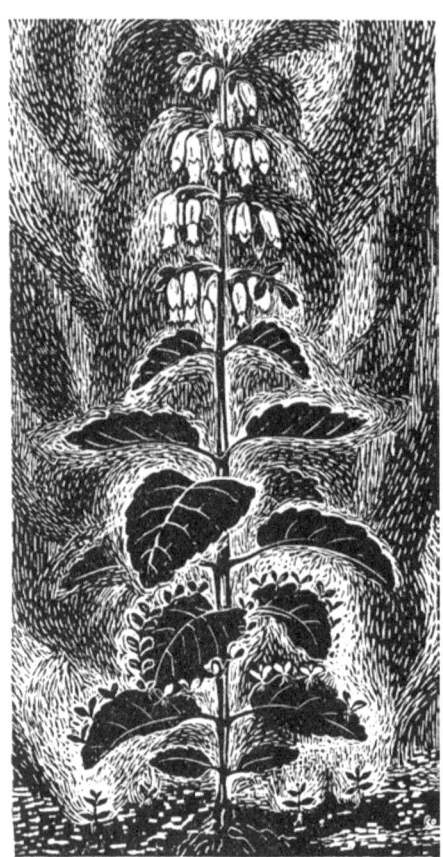

tures as high as 40°°F. Due to its strong vitality Bryophyllum was once used as a remedy for wounds and other ailments. Rudolf Steiner recommended it for conditions where outer processes are not sufficiently warded off by the lower human organization which works against the forming, shaping upper organization with overly strong and subordinate forces. Then the etheric body becomes overly powerful and rampant in this region and the organizing forces of the astral body become too weak. Here we have a primal form of disease which Rudolf Steiner called "hysteria" whereby he meant something much more comprehensive than what most people mean by this term. (He called the polar, primal form of this disease "neurasthenia", where there is a pathological predominance of the processes of the upper organization.)

Bryophyllum is useful as a soporific if the sleeplessness is caused by the condition described above, since healthy sleep is dependent upon a harmonious interaction of the etheric body with the astral body. On going to sleep the latter becomes separated from the upper organization that is the vehicle for consciousness and connects itself with the lower organization that is always in a state of deep sleep.

Sedum acre – stonecrop, wall pepper

Wall pepper thrives in desolate, sandy areas, gravely slopes, poor soil, rocky fields, gravely beaches, sand dunes, ruins, dams and on horizontal roofs that are covered with gravel, for it likes to test its great vitality by battling against crumbling rocks, whether they are siliceous or calciferous. It is the most vigorous species among about 150 others in the Sedum genus. Its strong, vegetative principle allows its creeping shoots to have many branches and to spread out into mats. The fat, roundish, needlelike leaves are crowded around the stems. Every torn off piece of shoot takes root rapidly and rocky fallow fields are quickly covered by luxuriant, green oases. Although the formative forces of the lower pole – life ether and

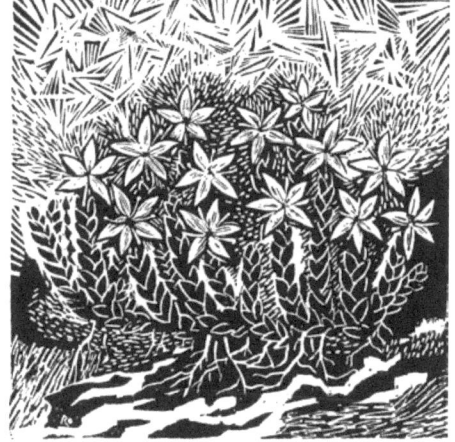

chemical ether – mainly live in such congested stem–like leaf formations, – the upper formative forces – light and warmth ether – soon do just as well. The terminal shoots with their many blossoms rise up out of the green islands with a strong, sunny golden luminescence around St. John's tide. In spite of all the congested succulence, the plant can connect itself harmoniously with an active flowering process and it can connect its strong etheric portion with the astral realms in an intensive way. A vigorous silica process that becomes manifest in a high silica content (36%) in its ashes is a big help in this plant.

This sedum species brings light and warmth processes into the mucilagenous, juicy vegetative organization in such an intensive way that it forms inflammatory, acrid, blistering substances. The herb contains sugar, fruit acids, resin and wax and also Vitamin C and rutin ("Vitamin P") which so often occur together. A deficiency in the latter leads to fragility of the capillaries in the skin and bleeding. One often finds the two vitamins mentioned in plants that vigorously overcome barriers to biological processes arising because of poor soil conditions (citruses, Rosaceae, Cruciferae, Sea Buckthorn) and that let themselves be helped by the cosmic forces that radiate in. Rutin shows this through its dye nature; it belongs to the widespread yellow dyes, the flavones.

The herb was used to make compresses for skin ulcerations and burns. The combination of a silicic acid process with a tough vitality that conquers dead soils, and the inflammatory principle that intervenes in the blood process enables this plant to have an invigorating effect upon the skin region, to attract the nourishing blood stream and to fire up metabolic activity in this area. Poor hair growth can be improved. Rudolf Steiner recommended this plant, together with others, for such purposes.

THE GOURDS – CUCURBITACEAE

Warmth processes that have been displaced into the watery realm

Just as a musically inclined person can liberate experiences of melody and harmony and the resounding proclamation of something spiritual out of her ear's sense perceptions, through which she "understands" what she heard, so someone who listens inwardly to a plant's forms and transformations can hear that it is identifying itself. Then we experience the motif and related themes sound forth which one recognizes as variations of the first one. Eventually the main theme occurs to us.

Just observe a cucumber or a squash throughout the year. Massive, luxuriant, juicy forms emerge from the seed with increasing force. A sculptor goes to work there might get some satisfaction from ponderous, crude and even monstrous things. As firm and tough as its branch is, it creeps back and forth along the ground obsessed with its weight, and it may lift itself up a little on a fence and try to attach its leaves and shoots to it, since it can't grow up straight by itself. Whereas in normal plants the shoot carries itself up powerfully against gravity and lets its new leaves spiral around something that is clearly perpendicular, the shoots in vines or climbers have no power to stand up and do not externalize the tendency to arrange leaves in a spiral way. Depending upon whether the main shoot or the side branches are taken hold of by the spiral tendency and they become either vines or climbers.

The juicy swelling that follows germination tells us how intensively water – the element of all sprouting – is sucked up by the growing plants. But this water does not become sufficiently light, it becomes congested in lower regions instead of flowing uphill, light and free, and arriving in upper, refined shaping regions. Mighty warmth forces work into the early stages of growth although their right time and place would have been in the formation of flowers and fruit. Brooding warmth forces prematurely and excessively take hold of the fluid, plastic part of the lower organs that still belong to the earth and water and make them blow up into gigantic, roundish forms at various places. In some cucurbits; it is the root, in others it is the stem, in most of them it is the leaves, in many it is the flowers and even the fruits. This is where we find the biggest fruits in the plant kingdom, that one can't even get one's arms around, weighing hundreds of pounds, and also fruits in which the rinds are pushed out into lumps, warts and thorns by the unstoppable, proliferating growth.

The plant's lower part greedily sucks in moisture and humus and it stuffs itself with watery earth to such an extent that the upper part cannot master and refine this coarse material and lead it up into the region of warmth and air in a worthy way in order to receive the cosmic gifts of the upper regions with ennobled organs. The lower part does not purify itself enough for the upper part. If this were to happen one would get a plant that was still massive and coarse, but one that stretched up into the air and the warmth – say like a sunflower. (Just convert a cucurbit into a sunflower in your mind and feel what would have to happen.) The plant turns to light and warmth just as greedily as to humus and water; cosmic things materialize, but matter is not sacrificed to them. The "material drive" outweighs the "form drive" by far.

Thus many blossoms form and they strive upwards and become sunny and bright colored; but with their odd, coarse forms they wouldn't do much for a bouquet, and they cannot emerge from a shadowy sea of leaves. Of course a lot of nectar flows into them. A tremendous growth that can spin over the biggest compost pile (stood on end it would be a tall tree!) finally swells up into the massive fruits that are brimming with sap and that bear a large number of seeds that are filled with oil that was created by warmth. The monstrous spheres do not really become ripe, they remain in a state that is between leaves and fruit, unfinished and not really cooked. One has to add sugar, acids and spices to cucurbits and cook them in order to make them artificially tasty and get them to the stage that apples, pears and oranges have reached by themselves.

The shoots' growth stops in spherical cucurbits like cantaloupe and pumpkins and if it continues one gets cucumbers and snake melons. The metamorphic forces that are otherwise mainly active in leaves in the plant kingdom are particularly active in the fruits of American, tropical cucurbits, which can take on the forms of bottles, umbrellas, bishop's hats, horns, fish and cones. The lower sculptor in a plant entity pushes liquids up into the warmth region of the fruits. Watery and warmth elements proliferate into each other and are not cleanly separated. One sees this repeatedly so it is a typical element in cucurbits. There are more species over in Africa and Asia – melons, bottle gourds, wax gourds (Benincasa) – which greatly intensify the wax formation impulse that is indicated on the outside of European cucurbits, Luffas (which extend the solid, fibrous part of the stem into fruits that look like cucumbers), and coloquints. The slightly bitter principle that is often found in our cucumbers is greatly enhanced in the latter. This bitter cucumber's leaves look like those on oaks, and their deeply lobed shapes disclose that a plastically swelling element is in a battle with a contracting, bitter one. Its round, smooth, yellow fruits are the size of apples. The fruit is flesh becomes terribly bitter, spongy and dry, as if it were dried out by the wind in the deserts near the Mediterranean where it grows.

The battle of the two principles becomes manifest in a different way in the squirting cucumber (Ecballium elaterium), which also contains a very sharp and bitter sap. The juicy swelling presses into the fruit and a bitter compressive element also presses in from outside. This produces a tremendous inner pressure; the ripe, pigeon–egg sized fruit separates from the stem with explosive force, and the seeds and the bitter, slimy sap squirt out up to 20 feet away. The fruit bursts in other cucurbits (Momordica, Cyclanthera explodans) and hurls the seeds through the air like in our Impatiens nolitangere.

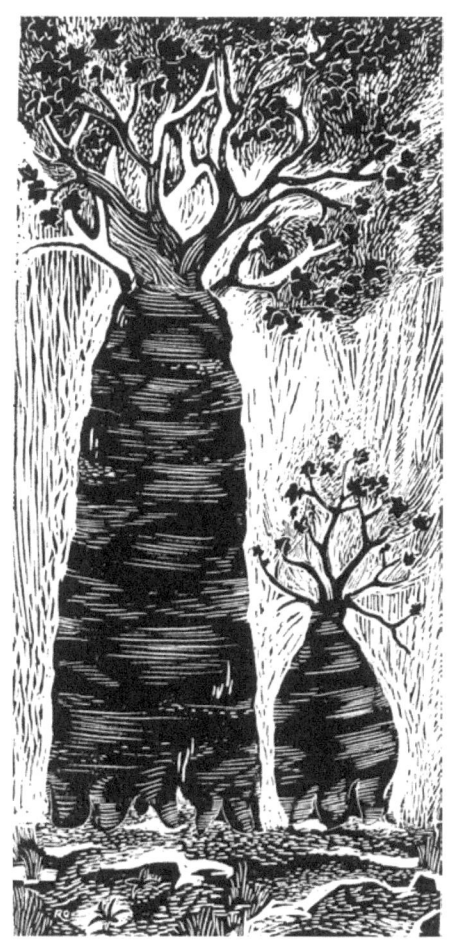

People often quote Rudolf Steiner's statement that bitter substances make man's "etheric body inclined to take in the astral body." The formation of bitter substances in the plant kingdom must be based on a corresponding process. In fact, cucurbits have to work hard in order to make their etheric, proliferating forces receptive to the impulses of the astral sphere which eventually draw forth from them quite an extensive flowering process. The permeation with bitter substances in helpful here.

The swelling forces which lead to cucurbits can get retained in the stem. Then one gets a peculiar variation on the basic theme, namely, Dendrosicyos, the only cucurbit tree which grows on Socotra Island in the Indian Ocean. A grayish white, soft trunk grows about 12 feet high; it is broad at the base and comes to a conical point at the top – like a giant, super-terrestrial Burgundy turnip, with grayish green, heavy branches coming out of its apex. Here a cucurbit becomes like a cactus, which is another possibility for this type.

However, the swelling tendency of the cucurbita can also focus upon the root and let it swell up in a monstrous way, which brings us to white bryony. If this process occurs in a dry, desert region, an enormously luxuriant, fleshy, swelling root can go down many yards while up above there's nothing but a leafless, thorny shrub, e.g., Acanthosyios, or Naras, which grows in sand dune regions in Southwest Africa. The predominance of warmth forces and the watery swelling process that has already occurred in the root region make it easy to understand why the fruits that grow above ground here are only apple sized; they are bright gray and the melon like flesh is particularly aromatic.

Another metamorphosis is in some forest plants, although only in the tropics, where in fact most of the 800 cucurbit species grow. The slight climbing impulse of our cucurbits is enormously increased in tropical forests; they climb and wind like vines up to the tops of the trees, where they lie heavily in the tropical sun and brood, just like they do on our compost piles; or they are like our bryony, which will climb up hedges and spread out on top of them in the light and air. On the whole, the species are lighter, more delicate and they gradually get rid of some of their earthiness on their long way up. Malayan Zanonia macroscarpa even drops winged seeds out of fruits as big as one's head which can fly a long way. Trichosanthes from Southeast Asia spins out its petals into tips. However, the basic cucurbit motif is recognized everywhere.

The main medicinal effect of cucurbit fruits is upon our metabolic system; the abnormally activated fluidic system becomes permeated by inflammatory warmth processes. The bitter resins and glycosides in coloquints and the dehydrated sap of squirting cucumbers (elaterium), speed up peristalsis and the elimination of body wastes, including urine. Excessive use can result in diarrhea, vomiting and bloody stools. However, white bryony, which goes through the fruiting process in its roots, has a polar effect on man's upper organization. It is the best healing plant in this family, and we will devote a special section to it. We owe two previously completely unknown applications of cucurbits to Rudolf Steiner. He recommended the addition of cucurbit flowers to calcium phosphate for a tendency towards rickets and malnutrition. In rickets one has a pathological interaction of the fluidic warmth systems. The I organization can not carry out the cooling processes which form healthy bones sufficiently; the rickettsial child's body is too watery and warm, as it were. There is a tendency for deformations here, since a harmonious human form is an expression of a normally functioning I organization.

From what was said above about the abnormal interaction of fluidic and warmth processes, connected with the deformation of fine, formative forces through a predominant material drive in cucurbits, one can see that the processes in them are comparable to those in rickets.

Whereas the I organization cannot control the warmth processes sufficiently in rickets in order to make healthy bones, it is hyperactive in the opposite way in sclerosis. Then it not only reduces warmth development for the skeleton but also for the vascular system and other organs. Rudolf Steiner recommended the use of a melon preparation here. Melons carry out their sugar process in the fruits much more intensively than squash or cucumbers do. If one separates off their watery processes and retains the finely organized solids together with all of the carbohydrates, one gets a substance that has an unhardened form. After all, as a tissue it held the fruit is pool of sap together so that it did not slosh around. The sugar gives this formative process a connection with the I organization.

Bryonia alba – white bryony (fence turnip)

The dusty, hot road was bordered by hawthorn hedges on its way through a sunny landscape based on weathered primal rock. Our attention was drawn to shiny, dark green, soft haired, delicate, cucurbit leaves that were held up by tendrils; a large number of little yellowish green flowers were visible and also many, little green berries that were beginning to get black. When one stepped behind the hedge into its northern shadow one could see that the soil which sent up this plant was loose refuse that was permeated by decomposing humus, to which the village dump nearby had no doubt contributed. Thin stems had shot up mightily, sending side shoots through the hedge, looking for light and warmth. However, the main mass of leaves had laid itself over the crowns of the hawthorn bushes and had spread out comfortably, and it was now enjoying the hot sun.

We decided to get the mysterious root that was once sought and used like the mandrake in northern lands. The moldy ground was soon dug up, and we were amazed at the mighty formation that the earth had incubated out there, which was comparable to a human torso with fat legs; it filled the wheel barrow with which we brought our find back home. Now a sharp unpleasant smell spread out, while hands that had touched the watery formation too much became red, inflamed and slightly swollen.

Here one could clearly see that Bryonia has practically finished its cucurbit formation in the root. The "water process" remains down below in the dark and heavy region. The monstrous, plump element is developed there. The root draws these formative tendencies away from the upper part of the plant. Thereby the upper growth became lighter and more delicate. The leaves, flowers and berries show this — just compare them with a melon or a cucumber. Warmth processes are pressed into this water process in a way that is typical for the whole family, but only manifested in the root region here

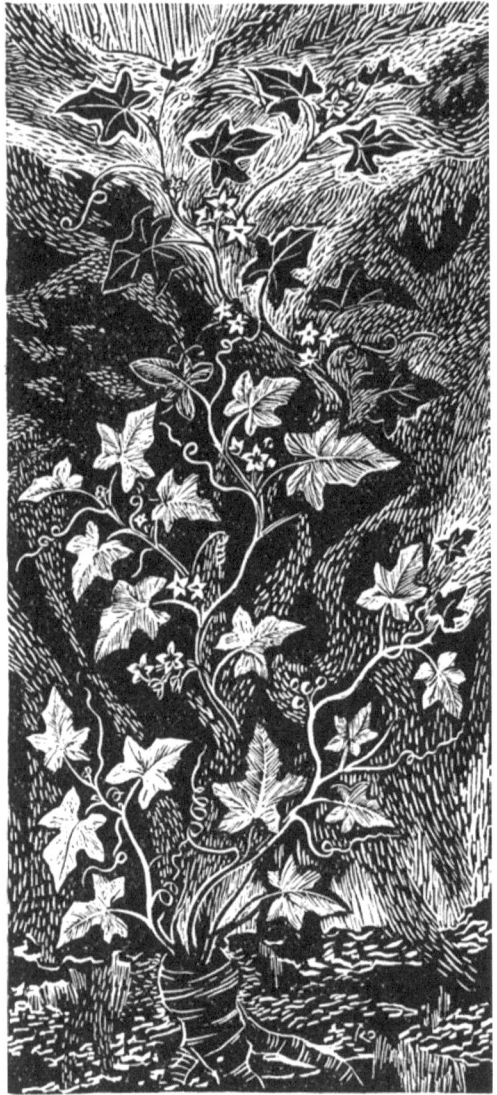

The effect of this plant upon man is displaced from the lower pole (permeation of the fluid system in the metabolic region with inflammatory processes) to the upper pole in accordance with the effects which roots have. One arrives at a pathological interaction of formative forces and members of man's being along the lines of a Bryonia process.

Man is made into a hedge turnip, as it were. In a healthy human being warmth and light ethers are mainly active in his upper organization and etheric body, and the chemical and life ethers are mainly active in his lower organization – the first pair more in the service of the I and astral body, and the second in the service of the physical and etheric bodies. But now a different division is aimed at; light and warmth ethers are driven out in the upper region and the chemical ether flows after them from below upwards, bearing excessive wateriness with it. The weakening of the warmth organization is disclosed by chilblains and shivering. The I organization no longer intervenes in it or controls it. The thinking activity that was excessively stimulated at first, gets tired; weak thinking and forgetfulness show that the I no longer fully controls the part of the etheric body with which it thinks (the part that is active in the head). A morose or lachrymose nature and vivid dreams indicate that the astral body is having difficulties with the physical body. The formative processes that proceed from the head become weak; teeth get loose and inflammatory swellings arise, like the ones that accompany and tonsillitis. Dizziness in the morning shows that the I and the astral body which have to come back into man's lower members have lost their conscious power over them. Congestions around the head and throbbing headaches arise. The metabolism shoots into the periphery too strongly and skin eruptions arise. Runny noses, eyes and chest sweating indicate that the fluid organization is pressing upwards too strongly.

Bryony is one of the "great" healing plants and is a powerful remedy for the treatment of various colds. The peculiar structure of its forces assures the experienced doctor that he can get quick relief with bryony when outer fluctuations of warmth and cold affect the system of nerves and senses to such an extent that the I and astral body no longer have full control over their warmth organization, when the lower cold fluids press upwards and are excreted due to the resulting disturbed equilibrium and when chilblains and fever accompany these various kinds of exudate in connection with rheumatic complaints.

Irises – Iridaceae

In this connection it would be helpful to the reader to look at the section on Liliaceae in Volume I of this work. Like the Liliaceae, the Iridaceae have an etheric congestion in their lower organs. Therefore they grow bulbs, corms and swollen rhizomes that are full of moisture; some species also are surrounded by moisture, growing on moors and in water. The shoot is held fast at this lower pole, often in a very shortened form; in many species the leaf formation is limited to a rosette or a mat on the ground. Shoot lines and leaf surfaces become fused, long grassy leaves that are often pressed into one vertical plane, spray out like a fan of lines, instead of the "normal" vertical line of a shoot, around which horizontal leaf surfaces circulate in a spiral. Once this congestion at the lower pole is overcome by the mighty flowering impulse, a flower stalk shoots up and develops its blooms. It holds the inferior ovary within itself and gives the lower, tubular fused flower parts some of its tendency to elongate. Calyx and Corolla are one colorful unity with its vertical tulip-like forms, but often also "throats or mouths" that tend towards the horizontal. The fusion of the lines and planes can also be seen in the flowers, where the pistil strives upwards linearly but often tends to be tripartite dividing into three leaf-like stigmas, which can arch over the outer petals like upper lips. This plant lives so intensively in fluids, and sends plenty of nectar upwards. The flower's hues have the transparency of water colors.

All of this tells us something about the special interweaving of water and light forces in the plant process. What one sees here in the living plant is something similar to what the elements reflect when they show the sun's image as a rainbow on a veil of silver drops against a dark background of clouds, and Iris the rainbow goddess appears with her colors.

Compared with the Liliaceae, the Iridaceae have become one degree more earthly. This is indicated by the inferior ovary that has slipped down into the stem, and also by the more intensive solidification processes in their subterranean organs, where one finds a lot of starch, and not just sugars, as in the Liliaceae. However, even here the formation of much mucilage keeps the lignification processes from becoming overly active. Bushes, trees or vines do not occur in this family.

Crocus, iris and gladiola are the three main forms our type takes on, as it brings the flowery element right down into the root region or near it. Over 1,000 light loving species live in the northern and southern tropics and temperate zones. South Africa and the Mediterranean region are full of them. We will describe two medicinal plants that are typical for the family, Crocus Sativus and Iris Germanica.

Crocus sativus – Saffron Crocus

Saffron thrusts its violet petals out of the earth in the late fall, just as meadow saffron (Colchicum autumnale) does and it has been cultivated in the Mediterranean region for ages. The root and corm formation springs directly over into the formation of flowers. This crocus celebrates the hour when the earth takes all of the presents of cosmic light and warmth that the stars streamed out to it during the summer and stores them deep down within it. The three fiery yellowish red branches of the style stand in the bright lilac perianth tube, almost like a flower or a bag of leaves themselves, very narrow grasslike leaves stand around this warm, spicy smelling flower. For all of its similarity to Colchicum autumnale, the sensory–moral impression one gets from the two is quite different. The magic colchi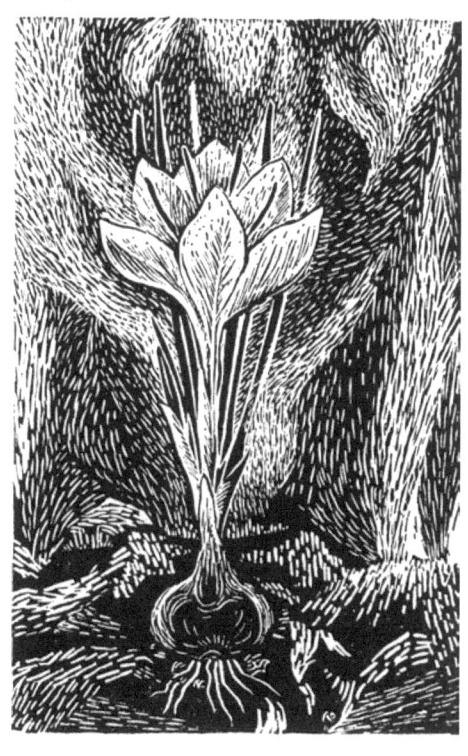cum herb belongs to the damp and cool element, whereas saffron belongs to fire and air; the former loves damp meadows, the latter likes sunny, rocky mountain sides.

(The signature of this plant is such that Rudolf Steiner pointed to the medicinal value of its corm and flowers. If suitably prepared, the corm combats swellings of the thyroid gland, just as Colchicum and cyclamen europaeum do (see the descriptions of these two plants below and in Volume I, and note the abnormal flowering times that oppose the normal annual rhythms of plants). The threefolding principle (see the first section in Volume I) teaches us that such an abnormal, congested formation can have a beneficial effect on the neck region. The dried stigmas from the blossom have long been used as a spice and a remedy for disorders in the sexual organs and other metabolic organs. Light and warmth processes have been powerfully interwoven into their fiery, yellowish red substances. They contain sugar, carotine and volatile oils that are closely connected with each other. The reader has already become acquainted with the dynamics of these substances from many descriptions of other plants, and will be able to sense the significance of such a natural mixture. It was recently discovered that very highly diluted, homeopathic doses of these work upon algae as "determination and fertilization substances", and that they mobilize their gametes. In man they drive blood strongly into the lower organs; severe inflammations, bleeding, miscarriages, lowering of consciousness and intoxicated conditions can arise; several grams of the drug can be fatal. The warming, stimulating effect of saffron upon the gastrointestinal tract was once greatly esteemed, and saffron was grown widely throughout southern Europe.

Rudolf Steiner showed how one can neutralize the harmful "excess forces" of the crocus' flowering process by combining it with antimony and corals, and he recommended this mixture as something that can have an ordering effect upon the whole blood process (Kalium Aceticum comp.).

Iris Germanica – German Iris

The leaf process of this iris sprays out of last year's tautly swollen rhizome and its long roots like a vertical, flat fan of sword blades; but this description remains an external picture if one cannot feel that a sword form is a metamorphosed lance, where the shaft and the blade of the lance are fused from the ground up. The sprout line and stem of the leaf in which the enlivened fluid streams "uphill" in the plant, and the leaf blade in which this fluid spreads out like a sea to the light and air, – both of these are a unity in irises right from the beginning. In addition, all of the leaves are united into a fan of swords as if into a single vertical leaf.

Such a formation belongs to both water and light, and yet both of these attack the earth-root pole strongly, and the latter firmly pulls towards it what would like to sprout upwards, unfold in the horizontal plane and circle around the upright element. The iris flower climbs out of the fan of swords, first as a flat, compressed bud or like a spirally turned point of a lance, and then it opens towards all sides in space. Each blossom seems to consist of four flowers, since three white petals streaked with violet and a yellow beard along the mid rib swing out wide and downwards; each of them is arched over by a petal like stigma and each is covered by a kind of an upper lip. The three other lighter, violet petals bend up and inwards as in a tulip. A strange and unique formation that enables one to recognize any iris at the first glance. Bumble bees get the deeply hidden nectar that is produced in the three tubes that surround the style.

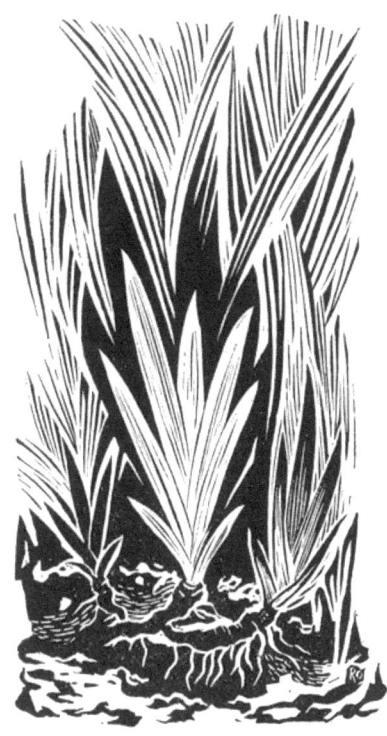

The flowers open around Whitsun. Each one blooms for a very short time and then slumps, softens and withers, but it is immediately replaced by one of the reserve buds. However, the high leaves that envelop each bud are dry as parchment. The fruit becomes a dry capsule, and as the fan of swords grows, desiccation processes are already taking hold of the leaf tips and their edges, so that the flowering process seems to suffer from a certain hyper-intensity in the plant's springing and shooting forces. The whole phenomenon above ground soon wilts and withers. Thereupon the subterranean life pushes a new joint out of the rhizome, which puts down its own roots and closes itself off with next year's leaf and flower buds.

The interplay of upshooting, juicy, plastic, fluidic, vital processes and wilting, withering ones that accompany the intensive development of flowers is a major motif in the Iris process. A strong etheric process

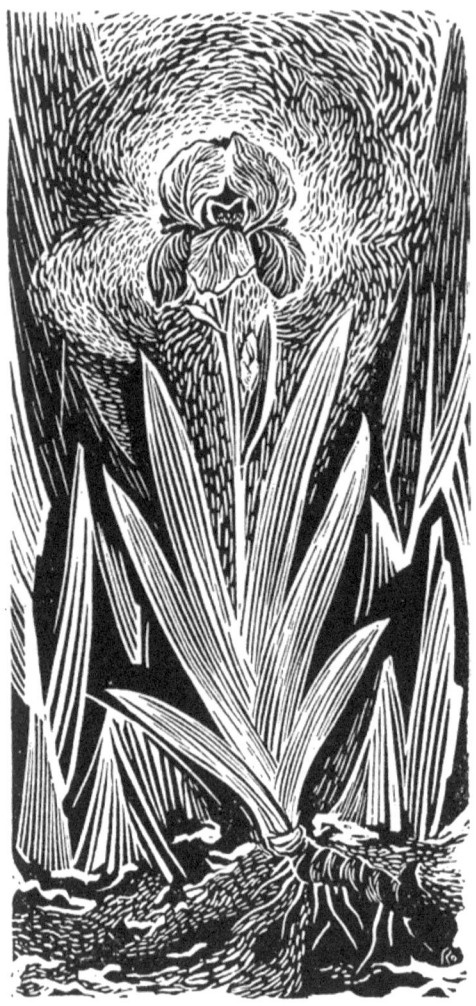

congested into succulence is fighting with an equally strong astralization process. Its powerful "etheric cushioning" prevents the iris from becoming a very toxic plant, but tannins and glycosides are formed, also substances that irritate the skin, although they disappear when the plant is dried, the poison motif nevertheless does sound through a little bit. Also one gets substances in the rhizome that smell something like violets – so the flowering process goes deep down, whereas the root element can be perceived in the flowers' dull and heavy fragrance.

The rhizomes also contain a lot of starch (about 50%), about 6% sugar, 10% fatty oils and a lot of mucilages, which are always present when something that is fluidic and alive protects itself against desiccation, hardening and lignification.

The formation of such substances points to the earthly–cosmic work of the plant's higher members and of beings in higher worlds upon the plant; hence such substances can stimulate the members of man's being in specific ways.

"Now in an iris we're dealing with something that has a strong effect on the I, as one can already see by its outer appearance. The repulsive smell and bitter taste immediately tell us that the I is interacting with the outer world in a strong and physical way. We have something in an iris root that stimulates this physical activity a great deal, namely, tannic acid. We also have something in it that work s upon the I's activity, starch. Finally we have something that has a physical effect wherever it goes, if it is stimulated to do so, we have resins in iris roots. All of this can make the I particularly lively and active." Rudolf Steiner said this in a lecture to doctors (*Anthroposophic Spiritual Science and Medical Therapy*, lecture 7) and he added that an I that is stimulated in this way can intervene in the fluidic organization, if the latter is in danger of falling away from its organizing forces, as in edematous conditions.

Therewith Rudolf Steiner is indicating the way in which man's highest member, the I organization, interacts with the iris process. Particular attention is paid to smell and taste. If one arranges the many smells in a spectrum and does the same with tastes, pleasant and repulsive smells will confront each other like opposite poles, and so will sweet and bitter tastes. Pleasant things dampen our consciousness and we lose ourselves in them, whereas we wake up and become more aware of ourselves when we oppose and reject things. When we taste food we feel how it gets fluid and how digestion takes hold of its inner qualities. We become aware of the beginning of this process with our gums and tongue, but we lose track of what goes further down inside us. We taste sugar's sweetness and the starch that is readily changed into sugar very intensively at the tip of our tongue; we can taste tart things like tannins and bitters further down in the regions where outer digestion passes over into the inner and to the re-enlivening that occurs after the food's own forces are destroyed. What has been liquefied in this way must be absorbed into one's own fluid organism – which itself is entirely enlivened fluids – where the liver is particularly activated by bitter substances.

Where the sense of taste permits us to participate in everything that takes place in the plant between fluids and solids and between etheric and physical things, smell leads us into a realm where volatile things become separated from plant juices and where airy things can be shaped but not held fast. We have often mentioned that the way that extracorporeal astrality takes hold of the plant's etheric organization becomes manifest in its fragrant substances. The kidney system in man brings his astral organization into his fluids and etheric body, and the essential oils that are the carriers of aromas have a stimulating effect upon it. (The volatile oil process becomes more physical in the formation of resins and it undergoes a certain solidification.)

Thus remedies from iris rhizomes can draw the I more strongly into the perceptual activity of the metabolic region; the enlivening processes occur in accordance with the I. All fluids can be permeated by the etheric body and also by the I's power. (In edematous conditions the etheric body is unable to enliven all the fluids sufficiently; they become dead to some extent and get stuck in pockets, in the realm of heavy, earth forces.) However, remedies from irises and some other plants stimulate the kidney process to excrete the fluids that can not be vitalized sufficiently and that become a foreign body for the organism.

The human I organization permeates the fluidic organization with warmth, light and levity and holds the body upright. The sunny forces of a spiritual, I element also work through plants along a vertical line that goes between the cosmic spheres and the earth's center. The plant saps of irises rise and fall in a particular way along this line. They are congested in the earth region. Then they become permeated by light, and they rise lightly up through the fan of leaves and through the flower stalk. After touching the astral zone that is revealed through the flowers they take the aromatic process and fall back down into the roots, leaving the upper regions without fluids, and thus shrivelling rapidly. The whole plant devotes itself to this rising and falling, congesting and shooting, swelling and radiating, as it shapes itself. The water in the iris process undergoes vitalization process and becomes physical. Water that has become physical is no longer held fast by its life process and so it vaporizes, dries up and drips out. It is with good reason that the word "physical" occurs so often in the short Steiner quotation above; the I is supposed to interact in the right way with the physical things in the fluids with the help of iris substances.

Another indication that we owe to Rudolf Steiner is that suitably prepared iris rhizomes have an effect on the swelling and tension condition of skin tissue, or on its "juiciness".

*

GRASSES – GRAMINEAE

The Formation of Starch in the Force Field of the Silica Processes

Forests and meadows or foliage and grass, make it clear that the whole earth's surface is a living place. Plants have gained the power to spread their kingdom over the earth's soil almost without a gap through these two forms of life, and to make the earth into a green star of life.

Therefore we will devote a few pages of this book to meadows and cultivated fields, and the plants that are on them. Most field and meadow plants belong to one large family—the grasses—which has a particularly long sub-family, the sweet grasses, with about 4,000 species. What power enables this plant family to take hold of certain regions on earth so completely and exclusively, to push all other plant life into second place and to flood green oceans over whole lands?

A meadow is a place of light, damp, fresh ground, and a breeze that blows over it freely. Its soil has root growth through it in all directions to such an extent that it belongs to the world of plants just as much as to the mineral earth; it lies upon the latter as a layer of sod, like an independent geological formation. The ability of grasses to connect themselves with the earth in such an intimate way is one of their main characteristics. Once a grass or a grain seed has gained a foothold in the soil it puts down some strong roots into it. The shoot sends out side shoots as soon as it gets to the first node and moves higher towards other nodes, or it sends out runners towards all sides which put down roots and send up new shoots. Thus every stalk becomes a cluster or a sword and even quack grass or other weeds in this family, that proliferate endlessly and can hardly be controlled, are only exhibiting the beneficial, ground penetrating root power that is a virtue of all grasses in a one–sided, excessive way. Depending on the way this multiplication occurs in the part of the grass that is turned towards the earth, a grassland is distributed and closes up without a gap, or wheat is lined up in rows in wide fields, or one tuft of grass shoots up next to another, as in New Zealand tussock pastures or one gets the clumps of grass that grow alongside South American or New Zealand waters or the clusters of bamboo stalks that shoot up from a single plant.

The superterrestrial part of the grass type is a condensed ray of light, a completely linear formation. A narrow leaf haltingly separates itself from a jointed stem and ensheathes it for part of its length before it moves away. The leaves have no petioles; the stem principle is mainly active in the central support. The potential flower is lifted up in the tip of the shoot, and one then begins to get a certain division; spikes or panicles appear. The leaves covering the florets often like to stretch out linearly into long awns or beards.

Individual grass flowers are small and stunted. They have lost their colored sheaths; one will look in vain for sepals or corollas. The inflorescence or spikelet includes a number of these florets which are exposed to the wind when they come out of their glumes, lemmas and paleos, since they have no sheaths. They are really "created" by the air for the air. It is not the airborne insect or bird that carries pollen to the feathery, airy stigma and styles. The air itself, the bearer of astral forces (Goethean scientists of the 19th century sometimes called it the great world-animal) takes the clouds of pollen into its breath and blows them at those stigmas out of its sphere that is permeated by light, warmth and cosmic forces.

Even though their individual flowers seem to be without colors and aroma, the blooming grasses on an unmoved lawn or a forest meadow are rapt in wonderful, delicate colors. A corporeal formation with something of the transparency of rainbow colors, or something that is closer o colored air floats over the forest of grass stems with orange, rose and violet tones. Blooming grain fields have characteristic, albeit delicate aromas. However, color and fragrances seem to be pointless in such wind pollinated plants, since they don't have to attract any insects.

There is a secret hidden within grass flowers. For in grasses the flowering process is seated where it is supposed to be; it only takes hold of the plant after a suitable preparation. Roots, shoots and leaves are all developed properly and consistently. After a suitable preparation the plant moves out of the fluidic, plastic, lower region into the light and warmth region, where it encounters the astral sphere. The astral never overpowers grasses or presses into their etheric and physical bodies. That's why one encounters no poisonous plants among the well over 4,000 species of Gramineae. (The poisonous ergot on rye is not due to its grassiness but to a fungus that proliferates on and through it.) Thus grasses are about as normal as plants can get. Their flowering process is plentiful and strong; what individual florets lack in the way of a complete development is more than compensated for by their numbers in the composite spikelets. But certain forces and virtues are dispersed with; beautiful appearance and showy splendor are sacrificed. Just compare grasses with the caryophyllaceae and their leaves that are singularly close to the stem, but with magnificent flowers. The immense formative forces that flow into such a development of flowers are sacrificed in grasses and directed towards a different goal. They are the big foodplant family in earth existence. Their etheric nature is so strong that they partly enter and merge with the higher realms in animal and man, and they are permitted to help with the building up of the latter's bodies. The specific animal nature is kept away from their florets, but grass and grain is given to animals as food. The milk with which the thousand-breasted Demeter feeds men and animals flows out of the essential substances of Gramineae. Grain couldn't give us bread if it had flowers like clove pinks or gladiolas do. (Gerbert Grohman pointed this out in an impressive way in one of his nicest books, *The Plant*.)

The manifold grazing animals live on grass. Each continent with its grasslands has produced particular kinds of grazing animals. Just think of the prairies and pampas in the Americas, of the buffalo herds that once filled North America, of the mountain pastures of all continents with the llamas, sheep and goats, of the steppes with their antelope and kangaroo species, and of all the horses on the broad Asiatic steppes and pastures. What a close interaction between plants and animals! Grass seeds, however, attract grain-eating birds, rodents, mice, and hamsters.

The grains are the staple foods for mankind. Where would our daily bread come from without them? Bread is the most human form of all foods; the human formative secret is inoculated into it and the whole way it is prepared. Grain is the only plant type that is capable of receiving this inoculation. Its nature can be absorbed by human nature through the preparation of bread.

Once the plant has been brought out of its condensation in the solidity and hardness of the seed by watery fluids and it begins to sprout and shoot, it opens itself to light and air, connects itself with the airy element completely in its blossoming, and as it ripens it experiences a permeation with cosmic warmth to such an extent that it dries out completely and it concentrates its life entirely on the spikelets. The bread preparation adds a series of four processes to this development in four stages, and with the same rhythm. First the solid grain is converted into meal by grinding, and this is converted to dough through the addition of fluids, which is subjected to the plasticizing forces of kneading. This is followed by an intensive creation process which loosens the dough and makes it porous, and then comes the warming and maturing in a baking oven. This gives rise to a food that is appropriate for the whole human being and for the way his members are fit together. For he bears solids in his physical body and he permeates his fluids with the body of formative forces or etheric body, the inner sculptor in his system. He aerates himself with his air organization that his soul or astral body moved into, and he lives in his warmth system with his spiritual member or I. Thus the breadmaking process has taken its measure from the human being. And the constitution of grain makes such a process possible.

The Gramineae's whole shape is created by a strict uprighting force. Grain that is knocked down soon rights itself again. In the rosemary section in Volume I we mentioned that the sunny, cosmic I nature of plants works through the vertical growth axis. The fact that the staple foods for the erect human being on the earth come from the grasses, or from that plant family that chooses such an extremely vertical growth line as its main shaping principle, is one of the gestures of earthly existence that tells one a great deal. The spirituality of the Gramineae becomes manifest in such a gesture. What is modestly left unspoken through the renunciation of flashy flowers is expressed in a higher sphere of existence in the human being.

> *It is not the bread that nourishes, what feeds us in the bread,*
> *is God's eternal word, is life, and is spirit.*
>
> Angelus Silesius

The Gramineae type is capable of much transformation; it has developed well over 4,000 species out of itself that grow all over the earth. The form of each of these tells one something about the kind of soil it is growing in and the conditions of light and warmth around it and about how the cosmic world is irradiating it. Cirque meadows, North Sea islands, marshes and swamps, dry and wet fields, rocky mountain slopes, river banks, ferns and bogs, reedy seashores, the Argentina pampas and North American prairies, steppes with camel grass and elephant grass, salty dunes and village clearings in the forest primeval – all have their particular kinds of grass.

And yet in spite of the many variations the basic motif is strictly adhered to. In all cases a grass plant remains a spear of light thrust into the ground and taking root there, if my readers will allow me to use this image, for it would like to express the secret of this plant family in the briefest way. The formative principle of grasses needs very few materials to develop all kinds of shapes. (However, it is impossible for grasses to create two forms: cactuses and vines. We feel confident that the reader can figure out why.)Thus every continent, zone, and climate on earth has produced its particular kind of grain. This shows one how sensitive the Gramineae type is to the earth's nature at any particular point and to the formative forces that are present there. Rice has a loose, light and airy nature. It reflects the light power of eastern lands and it gives their people a staple food. The top soil that is plastically saturated by water and is artificially preserved from too much earthly hardening must be prepared to receive rice seedlings with loving care; its cultivation amounts to a kind of hydro–agriculture. On the other hand, corn is the largest kind of grain and the one that has become most earthy.

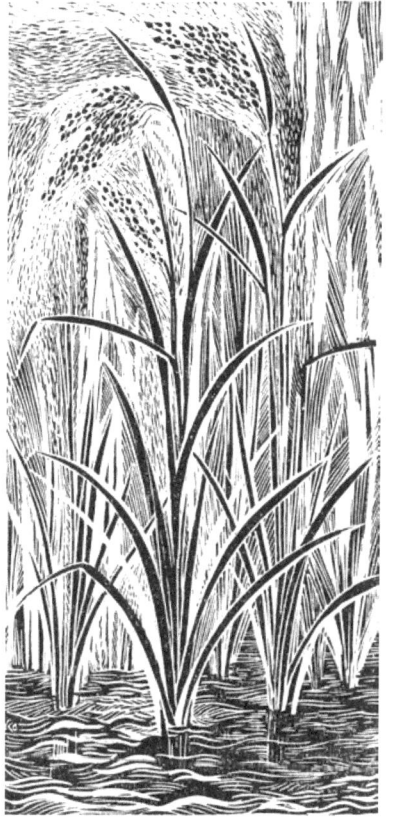

It is a gift of the western earth and its female ears that are contracted into plump, massive cobs further down on the stem show what kind of formative forces are in it. Here we have heaviness and coarse substances.

Rye, the grain that can stand the greatest cold and which goes relatively high up into the mountains, and towards the polar circles, tells us about the long light–filled summers with their cosmic forces that shorten nights around St. John's tide.

Species of millet are Africa's staple grain, especially in subtropical steppe landscapes. They are course, high and broad-leafed, and their influences fluctuate between panicles and cobs. One makes porridges and pancakes out of these grains from the east, west, south and north, but they are not too good for making bread. One can only really make that most human food, a loaf of bread, from the rye and wheat that originated with the peoples in the middle. The Graminea type takes in the four cardinal points that are imprinted in the earth's shapes or the world cross that is inscribed in them – as a life-shaping motif. This type listens to the conversations which the sun and earth have with each other through their formative forces. That is why the myths of all cultures and peoples tell us that the grains are a divine gift of the heavenly father to the earth mother. Sowing seeds was a cultic deed and harvests were also accompanied by cultic rituals. Just as the sun shines on all peoples, so it was given to Christians among all of the earth's peoples to feel heavenly forces in their daily bread, to eat it with reverence and to feel the divine power who not only was in the heavens on the sun but who descended to the earth and walked through Palestine's wheat fields with his apostles and united himself with our earthly bread and raised the act of eating into a sacrament. Even though wheat came from Persia and other eastern Mediterranean lands, it is the grain that could come down to all peoples and spread out to all continents. That is its solar blessing.

*

The Gramineae's greatest achievement is their organic synthesis of carbohydrates. The marvelous way in which the forces of the earth and sun communicate with each other and make starch out of water and the carbon dioxide in the air, and of how sugar is made from this can be seen particularly well in grains. After all, a ripe spikelet of wheat is practically nothing but a stem and an ear, in which the seed that was sowed reappears sixty fold. All of the plant's forces are directed towards the production of bread. Sugar flows towards the spikelet and it gradually solidifies to starch in the kernel. In sugar millet and especially in sugar cane this sugar process that flows upwards is stopped before it gets to the transformative zone of the floret and fruit region.

However the Gramineae's mighty carbohydrate process does not suppress the formation of substantial amounts of proteins and fats, so that one has a harmony of all of the basic food materials here which one can hardly find to the same degree of perfection anywhere else in the plant kingdom. Vitamin researchers confirmed this perfection in their own way. That is why one can make bread into a staple food and even into a food that is almost sufficient by itself, if one prepares it properly and does not destroy any of the grains' qualities. Rudolf Steiner gave far–reaching indications about this. He also advised that bread be made out of the four main European grains – wheat, rye, oats and barley and that one should add a few nuts to the dough.

Starches are not all the same; the kind that is generated in the Gramineae process has its particular virtues. This is due to the sunny nature of the type, which has connected itself with the earth realm in such a powerful and loving way. The starch in a potato tuber must be looked upon as much more one–sided and imperfect than the kind that is in grain kernels. When one begins to read in the world of formative forces or even begins to recognize the letters, one can arrive at such judgments by reading the biological phenomena. The night shade type can never attain the virtues of the luminous Gramineae type.

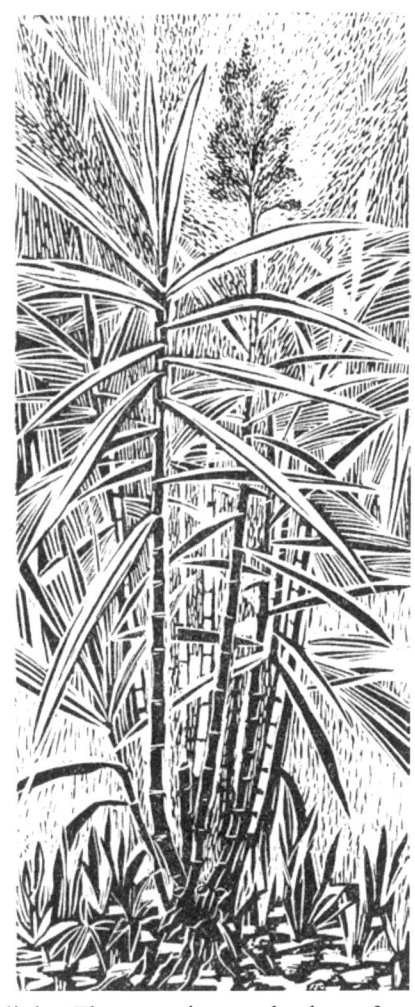

*

Radiant luminescence becomes manifest in this type of grassy plant in a particularly pure way. The type becomes able to incorporate this luminescence through something that can be called a mineral that has become light. The attentive reader has often encountered it in this volume on healing plants, and it is showing up again here in a particularly significant way. Grasses are among the plants that have the most silicic acid or silica. Some of them have as much as 90% of it in their ashes – especially in the bracts (glumes, lemmas and paleas) around the fruit. The seeds also contain considerable amounts of it. An awned ear of barley or rye is like an image of these radiating silica forces.

A wonderful synthesis of metals, present as trace elements, points to processes that stream in out of the cosmos and into the formative forces body or etheric organization. We refer you to the section on vitamins, below, for more details about the trace elements. Grains contain traces of iron, cobalt, nickel, titanium, copper, zinc, barium, lithium, and non-metals like boron, iodine and fluorine. For instance, millet is a grain that contains a bit of fluorine.

*

The proper management of silica is a particularly important aspect of forming, gardening and the cultivation of plants. Our many references to the silica process have made it ever clearer that we are dealing with a basic process in earth existence that is essential to life. Most of our earth consists of silica and silicates; silicic acid permeates all life and traces of it are present in our atmosphere and hydrosphere. Rudolf Steiner pointed out that plants would be shaped quite differently if our earth's silicic acid process was not so intensive. They would develop a blown up, cactus like, bloated growth that would lack fine formative forces. "Grain forms would look quite cosmic, the stalks would become thick and even fleshy at their lower ends and their ears would degenerate." (Whereas if the limestone process became too weak there would be nothing but creeping and climbing plants whose flowers would be sterile, and no food would be created.) Now these two kinds of plants do exist, as strong deviations from normal plant life, although they are not quite as extreme as the ones just described. The cactuses in the deserts and vines in the jungles are such aberrations. But grains and grasses stay away from these extremes. There are no succulents or vines among them.

Rudolf Steiner went on to say that certain forces work out of the cosmic periphery into earth existence through silica processes and others through limestone. The outer planets, Mars, Jupiter and Saturn, work through silica, and the heavenly bodies that are closer to us and the Sun, Mercury, Venus and the Moon, work through limestone. The plant's reproductive processes are promoted by limestone and the inferior planets, whereas the production of food stuffs is promoted by planets further away from the sun. "The siliceous element opens up the plant's being, out into distant world spaces; and if the plant being's senses awaken in such a way that they take in what the planets develop out at the periphery, far away from the earth, then Mars, Jupiter and Saturn are involved, whereas what enables the plant to reproduce is taken in from the Moon, Venus and Mercury." Water (whose connection with the moon's activity is shown so clearly in tides) mediates the forces of the latter planets to plants, whereas atmospheric warmth makes the forces that are mediated by silica particularly active. How strongly the first kind of forces affect plants depends upon how warm the air is, and air has a homeopathically diluted silica content in any case.

Vernal and sprouting forces are connected with the water born and calcium mediating forces of the moon and the inner planets; summer and maturation forces are connected with the warmth born and silica mediating forces of the outer planets. The grain species that are intensively connected with the siliceous substances, warmth and the cosmic forces of Saturn, Jupiter and Mars are able to create nourishing substances that are the basis of all human nutrition. And in fact, the grass type is something unique in the plant kingdom.

The plant's silica process opens it up for the sphere of cosmic light and warmth. It intensifies the leaf process that digests light, and it enhances the maturation forces and the quality of the food that is formed in the fruits. Following an indication by Rudolf Steiner, biodynamic farmers have been using a very finely diluted silica preparation as spray with great success. This complements the nature of grasses in a particularly fine way.

We will now direct our attention to another process in the Gramineae. Everyone remembers the sweet aroma of freshly cut swatches of grass and of dried, good, field hay. Although grasses have renounced beautiful, fragrant blossoms they can nevertheless form aromas. The wilting process brings them out. What appears here in a delicate way is intensified in the creation of very fragrant substances in tropical and subtropical bearded grasses. One often gets stems and leaves that smell something like lemons and roses as in citronella grass, lemon grass and palmarosa grass. Vetiver oil, from the root of Khuskhus grasses, has a pungent and heavy fragrance. Thus the type definitely has the capability of developing aromatic substances. But it suppresses it and doesn't allow it to stream through the flowers and into the outer world. Nevertheless, one should know about this side of grasses. It only develops in the tropics where the cosmic element is drawn into the earthly sphere so strongly, and where the terrestrial also proliferates up into the cosmic realms. Lignified, giant bamboo grass is an example of the latter side of tropical life, and the rush grasses of the Asiatic tropics are an example of the former.

The Healing Qualities of the Gramineae Type

At first glance one wouldn't think that the large food family among the monocotyledons and the giver of our bread would have anything to do with disease, but only with blooming health. And yet one associates one stubborn disease with grasses, and that is hay fever. Springtime, the time when grasses and grains blossom, is a time of almost unbearable suffering for some, and a time of discomfort for all those who have this disease. However, the fact that only relatively few people get it shows that it is a matter of predisposition and of a particular constitution. Only those who have the latter become hypersensitive when Gramineae bloom.

Rudolf Steiner explained the secret of a predisposition for hay fever, and he developed an effective remedy out of his insight into the nature of this disease. Hay fever is only the last phase in a process that already began in childhood as an "exudative diathesis", where the fluidic system and therewith the etheric body become too strong. Thereby the form giving higher members that develop the sense organs and the organs of consciousness, – the I and astral body – work too weakly and don't intervene in the physical and etheric bodies enough. The organs of the upper and higher members of man's being ("upper" because they are mainly active in the organs that bear consciousness in man's upper organization) become flooded by the overly active fluidic system. This makes these organs hypersensitive to outer stimuli and it results in a tendency to get colds and related diseases. The metabolic processes in those who have a predisposition for hay fever work too strongly from inside the organism towards its periphery. Now if one has similar processes in nature in the spring, when watery life unfolds in a mighty way and one has growth that shoots out centrifugally and loses itself completely outside, as one can see very plainly in the grasses' flowering processes – in other words, if the whole of nature gets a watery diathesis and then a kind of hay fever, the people who have a predisposition for a similar kind of thing cannot keep this overpowering nature process away from their bodies sufficiently. They become hypersensitive to all of the stimuli that are pressing into their noses and other sense organs. Their sense organs are taken hold by this inner organization, and they are unable to elaborate the processes in the outer world, to which they are opened, objectively enough.

Thus the Gramineae are not to blame for this disease—it is an already disordered constitution that is responsible.

This large plant family does produce a few medicinal plants (surprisingly few though). Their healing virtues are comprehensible from the type's features. Its main feature is the interaction of the silica process with the process that forms carbohydrates, which are both placed very strongly into the plant's vertical, cosmic–I line. The I organization is the member that is particularly active in the elaboration of starches and sugars. The silica process reinforces formative forces in the vicinity of all organs that serve the development of consciousness and self- consciousness.

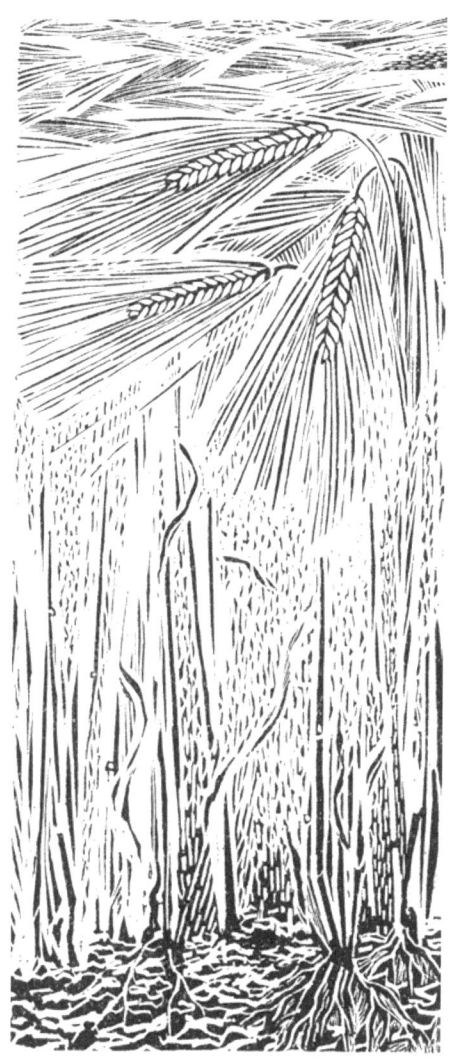

Baths and packs with decoctions of rice, oat straw, hay flowers and pollard enable one to get silica on the skin and through the skin. Such plant extracts and the silica in them enables one to heal and cleanse a skin that has become sick through a deficiently carried out silica process. Rudolf Steiner also recommended the use of ground and potentized barley awns in the treatment of sclerosis in old people, and this is difficult to understand unless one looks at the entire barley process. Barley is particularly active in the metabolism of carbohydrates. First it fills its kernels with starch, and when they germinate it does a particularly good job of transforming the starch into honeylike, dark, aromatically sweet malt, which is such an excellent nutrient and strengthening substance for convalescents. Barley ears produce particularly long awns; the silica process literally sprays out in the latter.

In this work on medicinal botany we have repeatedly pointed out that silicic acid tends to recharge a hyperactive sensory, nerve system and to increase its outer and inner ability to perceive things. However, it also has an extensive effect upon the relation that must exist between the I and astral body in order to secure the health of the whole human being. (One can regulate the relation between the physical and etheric bodies with remedies that contain calcium, and the relation between the etheric and astral body with antimony and with metals in general.) [9]

The relation between the I organization and astral body that should exist in healthy aging is disturbed in sclerosis. The I organization that has become too weak leaves the direction of breakdown processes to the astral body, which now is excessively active, and not in the way that the I organization would do it. Excessive mineralizing and hardening occur at the wrong places. For healing to take place the breakdown processes must be brought back under the control of the I organization, and the excess salt that has formed must be excreted. When the barley plant condenses sugar into starch as it is forming its fruits, it drives the excess silicic acid out into its awns and therewith also the excessive formative and hardening forces.

Homeopaths have used potentized corn cobs as a diuretic, to combat the formation of kidney gravel, and as a remedy for edema. This can be looked upon as an effect of silicic acid. The medicament is obtained from a "female" flower and will tend to affect the metabolism and lower organization. Here one should note that the silicic acid is kept in a plastic, living state, and is not excreted in an almost rigidified and mineral condition.

Oat preparations lead one over from purely nutritional food to healing food. Oats, the airiest and most light-loving grain, came from Europe. It has taken the radiant element that one sees in barley awns into its long pedicles and peduncles and thereby it has broken up the compact ear form into an airy panicle.

---

[9] See R. Steiner, *Polarities in Health, Illness and Therapy*, lecture 8.23.23, Penmaenmawr, Mercury Press.

This taking hold of the airy region occurs in a very watery plant here. Barley is the "driest" grain, which needs the least water, but oats likes moisture and exhales it into the air through broad leaves. Its juiciness makes it suitable for silage; it is like a cross between grass and grain. Barley grows in dry Mediterranean countries, whereas oats belongs more to cooler, northern mountain countries which have a lot of rain and longer days.

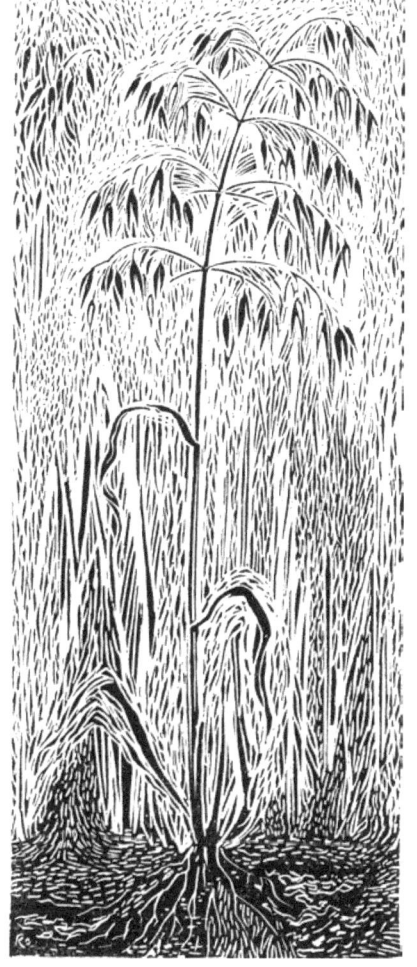

The interweaving of airy and watery elements that is peculiar to oats also becomes manifest in its saponin content. (For more details, see the entries under saponins in Volume 1 and in this volume).

The nice way in which oats elaborates the region of light and air can also be seen in a particular property of oatmeal. It contains substances which keep oils and fats from getting rancid through the attack of the air's oxygen. Oats can do something here which is done in the human organism through the activity of the astral body that works in our air system. Rudolf Steiner tells us that this member keeps the fats in our body from getting rancid. Likewise the etheric body keeps our proteins from rotting, and the I keeps our carbohydrates from fermenting.

A tincture of blooming oats has a regulating effect upon the relation between the etheric and astral bodies, because of its connection with the interweaving of fluids and air; it calms one and induces sleep and thereby promotes anabolic processes. Oat mucilage alleviates intestinal disorders that are connected with diarrhea, where the fluidic system has slipped away from the control of the astral body that is active in catabolic digestive processes.

Diabetics can tolerate oat carbohydrates better than the ones in other grains. Diabetes is caused by a weak I organization. This becomes manifest in its inability to take hold of and direct the carbohydrate process. The cosmic light region that builds up oat plants creates a carbohydrate process that can adapt itself more easily to the intentions of the I organization than other species of grain can.

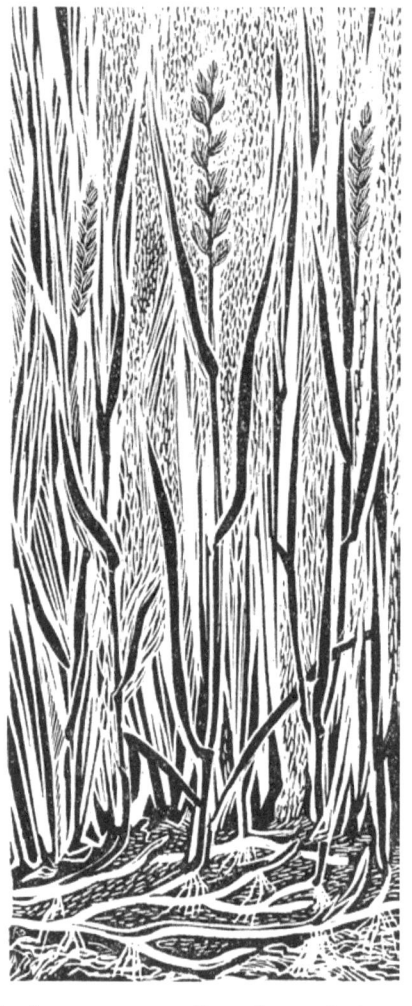

Couch Grass (*Agropyron repens* or Triticum repens) is somewhat similar to wheat, but it has placed its main biological thrust into its rhizomes, and thereby greatly exaggerates the power to produce the roots, side shoots and mats that belong to the nature of grasses. Couch grass practically makes tubers out of its rhizomes which it fills with carbohydrates, triticin and inulin and which it spices up with a little vanillin and volatile oils. They also contain saponins and a bit of silicic acid and iron. In homeopathy the potentized plant is used to treat inflammatory conditions in the kidneys and bladder, and for metabolic congestions. The roots have been used as food and as a component of remedies for liver disorders, chronic jaundice and gallstones. Its effect upon the carbohydrate organ, or liver, is an obvious one, the gallbladder process is supported in its outward direction.

Rudolf Steiner once recommended a salve that was to be made from triturated antimony and the juice from the root of quack grass. The idea here is that antimony and silica both have a special connection with the skin, and a corresponding effect on it.

Lolium temulentum, darnel also known as rye grass, or tares), is an annual, stiff–stemmed grass with narrow ears, and it is a very poisonous plant – which is something you wouldn't expect from a grass. But one stops being surprised at this when one learns that darnel has an almost imperceptible fungal process in it which spreads out its thick mycelium between the shell and adhesive layer of the seed. When the seed germinates, the fungus (endocomidium temulentum) grows along with the plant until it finds a place to spread out in the host plant, and its mycelium develops mightily in the flower's ovary.

This phenomenon then becomes connected with other parasites, with fungi that develop in the spikelets of grasses, take hold of their ovaries, develop a kind of nectar that attracts insects, and eventually grow into things that look like grains, are separated from the host plant, go through their own fruit development, and then attack the grasses flowers again. The best known fungus formation of this kind is ergot.

The intake of an extract from darnel seeds leads to a dizzy feeling, wooziness, visual and auditory disturbances, dryness in the mouth, inability to use one's speech organs, headaches, dazed feelings, states of confusion, trembling in the limbs, weakness and a desire to sleep. The body temperature drops and the heartbeat slows. The members of man's being that bear consciousness are driven out of the eyes, ears, organs of equilibrium and out of the experience and control of the outer world that is pressing in through the senses. The I's control over the instruments of speech and movement is also hindered. What one will have to see in connection with such disorders in the human organization is that what is abnormal is the uniting of the silica process in Gramineae with a fungal process. Fungi bear biological laws in them that belong to old Moon evolution, an earlier stage in earth's evolution. (For more details about this, see the introductory sections in Volume I.) No mineral world had developed at that time, and so parasitic fungi had to live on living things. Man's head development is connected with that of old Moon evolution. One could say that our head is placed upon the rest of our organization like a parasite. However our limbs developed during earth evolution towards the solid, mineral earth with its forces of gravity, etc. And our sense organs are permeated by fine mineralization processes; they are opened towards the outside world and they are meant for the perception and experience of the present–day earth and its mineral, physical aspects. Darnel drives man into behavior that is inappropriate for the earth in two directions, with respect to his sense organs and with respect to the limbs. It poisons the silica sphere in the human being. This sphere is "the physical foundation for the I organization". The latter "needs the silicic acid process down into those parts of the organism where the shaping and form giving activity meets the outer and the inner (unconscious) world." (Steiner, Wegman, *Fundamentals of Therapy*, Chap. 14, Mercury Press). Fungi darken this sphere. They benumb the senses and make one stagger.

*

The silica process becomes manifest in a special way in those most tropical grasses, the bamboo plants that shoot up so quickly. In some species silica becomes coarse, physical and earthly and it is secreted in dense walnut sized clumps as an inwardly grayish brown to blackish mass that has a white surface, in the hollow, lignified stems near the nodes. This product is called tabasheer, it looks like chalcedony when it is heated; it has been used as a remedy in the Orient for ages. One can expect specialized silica effects from a mineral that has arisen so directly out of a plant, a silicic acid formation that is secreted into a hollow plant stalk and not into a rock cavity or druse and has been released from the formative process and the vital dynamics of these very vigorous grass spades. The bamboo process is a plant process that elaborates the maximum amount of silicic acid, literally permeates itself with it, and secretes what is left over as tabasheer.

Arums – Araceae

Flowering Processes in the Root Region

The archetypal plant, that powerfully active being, with its harmoniously balanced "upper" and "lower" formative forces and its terrestrial and cosmic reference spheres, becomes characteristically distorted when it connects itself too strongly with earthly things and too weakly with cosmic ones. Then the lower organs proliferate and the upper ones shrivel. The growth congests into rhizomes and corms, the leaves spring directly from the subterranean sphere, and the flowers take too many earthy substances into them. If this earthly realm is a region with dark decomposition, rotting processes and brooding, putrefying warmth like the one we find in tropical forests and swamps, if the peripheral, cosmic forces only penetrate down to the ground in a weakened way, the being of the archetypal plant will be able to introduce arum plants into such regions. What brought the blossoms close to the congested root region in light–loving lilies and irises, but which left these blossoms with clear colors, fragrant aromas and nice forms, here becomes a grotesque, spotted, foul smelling plant and a fungus flower which often enough creeps into the earth or under water with only its upper parts showing. Carrion insects appear instead of bees; the floral parts develop a putrid odor and even get warm from the decomposition processes. Such flowers look like they've been animalized, and it is not surprising that the plants that produce them are filled with toxic substances. Spotty, dark colors play over the leaves, stem and uppermost leaf that sheathes the inflorescence. This leaf is often colored like a flower and it approximates flower forms with swellings like pots or spheres down below and a tubular bag above, but it is still only a leaf. Such spotty coloration always appears in plants when light and darkness work together in a chaotic way, and they don't unite in the harmonious and ideal way that one gets in green of plants.

The actual small flowers are arranged in spirals or whorls around the shoot that is like a rod or club, and which can wind itself around in serpentine spirals and often closes itself off with a blackish brown head, so that one might think that one had a mushroom wrapped in a greenish brown leaf. In *Irrwege eines morphologisierenden Botanikers*, (Byways of a Morphological Botanist), Goethe describes how a European botanist, who was sent such a plant from the tropics, erroneously thought that it was a new kind of mushroom.

In this work we have often pointed out that the earth's forces proliferate beyond themselves in the tropics (whereas cosmic forces take on an earthy tinge), and so there the type is tied to the dark earth and can climb up trunks for another ten feet and spread out Philodendron or Monstera leaves that can subsist on very little light, in the twilight of a tropical forest. The numerous roots that break out of the branches up in the air show that one is still in the earthy realm. For in the tropics the "earth" extends somewhat up into the airy region. That is why some plant families in the tropics have species that grow into trees whereas in the temperate zones they only have herbaceous species which at most have rhizomes under the ground. In arums the strong vitality of the root region pushes up above the earth's surface. In some species germinal corms form on the shoots; the feathery leaves on others fall off and form buds on the ground that send down roots and become new plants. Something of the vitality of a fern leaf becomes manifest here at the stage of a higher plant. One could call arums a synthesis of ferns and fungi in the realm of the flowering plants. The influence of an old animal–plant (lunar) principle can also be seen in the formation of milky saps in many arums. (See the many descriptions of milky saps in Volume I, and also about animal–plants and the old Moon stage of earth evolution.)

However, the type moves into brighter forest clearings in some species and unites itself more clearly with light forces. Here the spotty surface disappears, a dense mat of long stemmed, leafy shields shades the soil, and nutritious starch fills corms that are head size – such as Colocasia esculenta, the elephant's ear or dasheen of the Pacific Islands and southeast Asia, and Colocasia antiguorum, the taro of the Polynesians and one of their main foods. (Encyclo. Brit. 1979 under "Arales") One has to cook Arums in order to detoxify them. In Alocasia the starch accumulates in their bulbous underground stems.

When the type and its runners press completely into the open in the temperate zones, on the shores of lakes and ponds and in ditches, it resembles grasses or water lilies. Slim, narrow leaves and reedlike spadices shoot up; a spicy but still somewhat oppressive smell pervades the corm and upper parts of calamus root, or the spates lighten up into friendly colors, such as white in the calla lily (Zantedeschia aethiopica).

This more or less exhausts the number of forms which the arums can take on. Their nutritive value and beauty remains doubtful even in their best representatives. The motif of a distortion of the archetypal plant towards the "lower" pole tells us what we can expect from this type in the way of healing effects, namely, upon the metabolic processes in the head, senses and nervous system. We will look at two plants from this viewpoint, Lords and Ladies and calamus root.

Arum maculatum –Lords and Ladies

The whole shape of Arum maculatum seems to be bound to the subterranean sphere; fatty, waxy, green, pointed leaves that reveal their love of shadows through their brownish dark violet spots. The flower region looks as if one of these lanceolate leaves had wrapped itself around the flower spike like a bag, and therefore had been forced to act something like a corolla. Its green color fades, a whitish red tone appears, and often enough the dreadful spots reappear. The lower part of the spate (or leaf which becomes a sheath for the flower) encircles the blossom–bearing part of the rodlike spikes or spadix, narrows to a neck that is closed by a hairy net, and opens again into a leafy surface that discloses the bare, clubend of the spadix. Thus the flower is thrust into the leaf region and the leaves into the root region or into the stem that has been pressed together into a walnut sized corm. Around the beginning of May this flower unfolds in the decomposing leaves of beec h forests, or in any deciduous woods. Some of the brooding decomposition warmth seems to push its way into the fungous flower which has a carrion smell and a feverish warmth, with which it attracts flies. Once the small ones pass through the net they are caught, and they wander around the lower female flowers while the upper, male flowers drop pollen on them until the hairs on the net shrivel and the flies can escape. The flowers and leaves then wither so that in the fall only the spadix is left, encircled by a tight cluster of coral red berries.

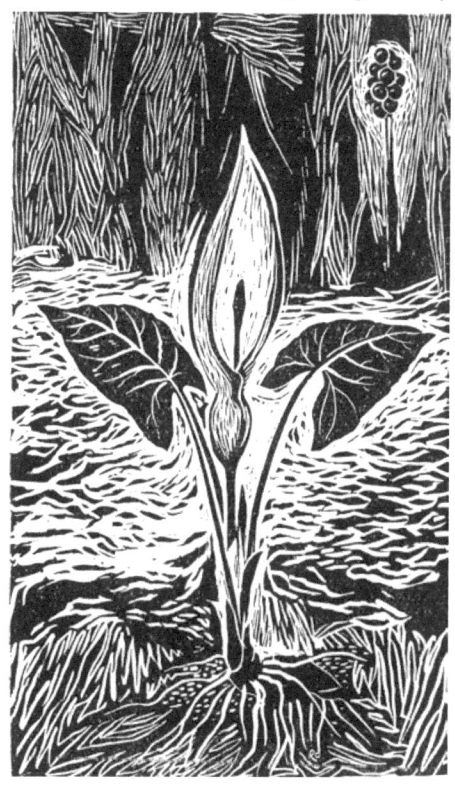

Farmers in many regions used to look carefully at this inflorescence in May, and from this they thought that they could predict how fruitful the earth would be or how good the harvest of their main crops would be in the fall. The female flowers that are grouped in close spirals around the lower end of the "rod" were supposed to tell one something about the harvest of root and tuber crops. The following sterile flowers, like hairy threads constituting the inner net or sieve, told them something about the first mowing, the following male flowers were connected with the fruit tree and grape harvest, the following outer net of sterile flowers like hairy threads was an indicator for the second mowing, and the club–like end announced the length of the grain harvest. Spots on the end of the spadix were supposed to indicate the storm frequency. However farmers used to look for prophetic indications about the coming seasons and their "deeds" in other plants as well; for instance, if elderberries bloomed especially well it was a sign of a cold winter ahead. Such views only seem strange to an age that has become estranged from nature. But anyone who can see not an accidental succession of 365 days but a living organism in the course of a year, a "timebody" that unfolds day by day "in accordance with the law that presided at its birth", like a plant, leaf by leaf, will not be surprised that the future is already there in plant life. A plant's etheric body is just as much of a time organism as its physical body is a spatial organism. Plant life with its interaction of terrestrial and cosmic forces is a copy of the year's life and it varies from one species to the next; a root can be called a wintry organ, a flower a summer organ, a leaf is vernal and fruits are autumnal. Arum maculatum with its special mixture of root and flower elements is sensitive to the way that winter and summer forces want to interact. The pistil in each flower is the last node in the rising stem, whereas petals and stamens are an expression of the encircling cosmic forces. One can tell how the forces of the roots and earth will interact with summer's forces in the periphery from the arum inflorescence with its individual flowers that are changed into pistil flowers down below and to staminate flowers above in one–sided ways. Just as farmers used to know and pay attention to their "lot days" on which the die was cast for a particular kind of weather for a shorter or longer period of time, so they looked upon certain plants as fortune telling plants for the coming harvest. The author has observed Arum maculatum flowers for many years and he can say that the old farmers knew how to read the book of Nature very well. It is not a matter of superstition in this case but of an intimate observation of nature.

    The attentive reader of this medicinal botany will not be surprised to learn that a plant is poisonous if its flower process presses down strongly into the root region. Araine is a poison that volatilizes through drying or cooking and which is concentrated in the roots but is also found in all parts of the plant. Here the astral region takes hold of the fluidic system and generates an airy, volatile poison, somewhat as in the

Ranunculaceae. Also there is a lot of oxalic acid in Arum maculatum as in many other plants which have to combat congestion. It also contains traces of cyanogenic glycosides.

As one might expect, the intake of the fresh root results in bleeding, swelling and inflammatory processes in the upper system. Rudolf Steiner recommended the addition of small amounts of the root's ashes to mouth washes and toothpastes, and he said that certain forms of epilepsy could be treated with a preparation of the fresh root plus bracken leaves.

In epilepsy the organs are constituted in such a way that it is impossible for the I and astral body to penetrate them; the activity of these higher members becomes congested at the surface of the organs, as it were. The attempts of the higher members of the human being to take hold of what is eluding them lead to epileptic seizures. Scientific research has established this. (See F. Husemann, *Das Bild des Menschen als Grundlage der Heilkunst*, The Image of Man as the Foundation of Medicine.) In Lords and Ladies it is clear that the coming cosmic participation (with astral and I elements) in its development is congested in the earthly participation in the same. The plant has to form its flowers without being able to raise itself into the region that is appropriate for this. The congested region of warmth and air in the ellipsoidal sheath around the inflorescence, and the numerous little animals that are attracted and imprisoned in it are a revealing image of the abnormal contacting of the physical, etheric realm by the astral–I realm. From this one can see that this arum root can address the epileptic process.

Acorus Calamus – Sweet Flag

If we step out of the shadowy woods with its damp humus soil and warm, decomposing leaves into the open air, to the boundary between pond and bank, we come to a place where the arum type finds quite different formative forces and conditions. It responds to this with a new plant; Sweet Flag. A long fleshy rhizome, up to two fingers thick, branches widely in a well watered soil. The sword–like, linear leaves grow up to 2 – 6 feet and have slightly wavy edges, with a touch of reddish purple near the ground; the stem and blade are fused into a unity. The terminal, three cornered flower stalk that bears the spikelike spadix also shoot up. But what a change from the Arum maculatum inflorescence! There is no sheath any-more, the spate is just a leaf–like extension of the stalk, and the spadix is out in the air and light. It takes quite a bit of practice in following the laws of metamorphosis before one can recognize the baggy pot of Lords and Ladies in the long green leaf, and the tightly arranged spirals of many, small flavors on the complicated Lords and Ladies inflorescence in the corresponding yellowish green flowers on a cob. The beneficial influence of illumined air, direct warm sun light and reflected light from the water has relaxed the whole plant formation, sent it up into the heights and permeated it with a spicy albeit dull aroma right down into the last root tip. The reddish berries only develop in its much warmer, southeast Asia home.

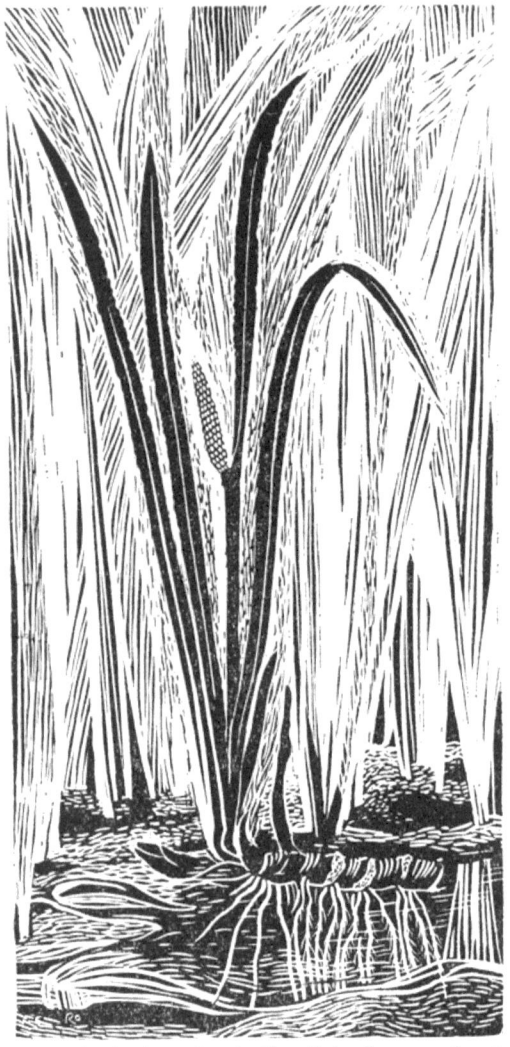

If we allow the material forces of Sweet Flag's vital formative forces we find a lot of volatile oil in the root (up to 3%) as the result of light and warmth forces, and also campherous materials, mucilages, tannins and a bitter essence that blends in well with the etheric oil. Medications containing calamus root tend to influence the way the I and astral organizations can intervene in the upper system, inflammatory processes in the mouth and stomach region can be combated and so can colics, lack of appetite and a slackening in digestive activity. Like thyme baths calamus baths have a good effect on children prone to rickets. The latter have overly watery constitutions, they cannot control their warmth activities via the I sufficiently and they cannot dampen them in the direction of a healthy development of bones and forms. However, Acorus calamus is a model for how warmth processes can become firm in watery environments.

Catkin bearers – *Amentiflorae*

We have often spoken about the overview of all the flowering plants which A. Usteri gave us that makes a magnificent process of unfolding and development visible. Usteri's system arranges the flowering plants into seven large groups, in accordance with the progressive perfection of their flowers. Although similar and related things are placed side by side, one doesn't get an advance in a straight line but a rhythmic return to a higher stage, just as after seven intervals the progressive tones on the scale lead to the eighth one which repeats the first one at a higher level. The chemical elements that are arranged according to their combining weights and valences show such great similarities after a number of them have been placed side by side, that the rhythmic repetitions can be put together in families and one comes up with a periodic table of elements.

Thus Usteri is the discoverer of a periodic system of flowering plants. He arranged them in seven large groups.

> Gymnosperms
> Proranales
> Ranales
> Monocotyledons
> Achlamydeae
> Archichlamydeae
> Metachlamydeae

The multicotyledenous, primal plants with naked seeds (gymnosperms) are the basic tone in this system or the prime in the scale of development; just recall the conifer trees which are the most important subgroups in the gymno sperms. We will look in vain for flower petals here. The shoot ends in a lignified cone and its spirals are similar to those of leaves. The scalelike carpels do not envelop the seeds yet. The development of color and aroma is minimal.

The flower form becomes more perfect in the Proranales and Ranales, the second and the third on the scale. The seeds are now surrounded by carpels, although the individual parts of the fruit are still separated and side by side. Many delicate, colored petals, stamens and pistils appear in a somewhat chaotic way, without strict, numerical relationships. But evolution hurries on to ever greater perfection in individual flowers, until the highest possible peak is attained in the fourth on this scale, the monocotyledons (one embryonic leaf). Just think of a flower on a tulip, lily or orchid that can no longer be made more perfect. A new beginning in this line of development is made with the achlamydeae, which now move towards another summit in the metachlamydeae via the archichlamydeae. At this high point for instance in the compositae, the whole inflorescence is brought to the highest possible perfection of form, as one can see in Edelweiss (Leontopodium alpinum), and not individual blossoms, for it would be impossible to get something that is more perfect than an orchid blossom.

Thus the achlamydeae (*a chlamys* = without a sheath) literally represent a new beginning. They can be classified into seven large subgroups, if one uses the principle of metamorphosis and enhancement as an ordering principle – the basic principle of all organic creation and shaping of life that was discovered by Goethe. According to Usteri these seven subgroups are:

(Sub Groups)	(Examples)
Piperoles	pepper
Urticales	stinging nettle
Amentiflorae	birch
Terebinthineae	wine–rue
Centrospermae	clove pink
Polygonales	buckwheat
Celastrales	grapes

A typical plant was named beside each subgroup to give the reader a concrete idea of the plants that are involved.

*

The catkin bearers or Amentiflorae which we are now going to explore can also be divided into seven families.

Juglandoceae	walnuts
Myritaceae	wax myrtle
Salicoceae	willows
Combretaceae Combretums	(tropical trees and shrubs)
Hernandiaceae	ovoid fruit trees
Fagaceae	beeches
Betulaceae	birches

The characteristic part of Amentiflorae is the inflorescence, the catkin, a hanging ament with flowers densely clustered around it, that either have no petals or only very primitive ones that are reduced to scaly bracts. The inflorescences are divided into staminate and pistillate flowers which are often found on separate plants ("male" and "female" ones). The catkin bearers are woody plants, either trees or shrubs. They take in the solidifying earth element in a powerful way, and they emancipate their biorhythms from the course of the sun by becoming plants that live for years. As the upper, outer shoots begin to produce catkins they work their way into the airy element which scatters the pollen and carries the insects that bear the grains to the stigmas. Winged fruits from willows, birches, etc. also glide back and forth through the air. Catkin plants bloom in the spring when Raphael–Mercury's breath blows across the earth around Easter time and the air gets into violent motion. Their home or main distribution regions are in the temperate zones, where winter goes over into spring in a vigorous way. Polar birches and willows extend far to the north. The new expansion of plants after the Ice Age gave catkin bearers plenty of room to become the main part of our deciduous forests, along brooks from the melting glaciers, at the edge of moors and in cirque fields, and in thousands of places along rivers. Earth, water and air are involved in their formation in a characteristic way and fire has less of a part. Catkin bearers like walnuts and myrtles have aromatic leaves, and others like beech and hazel nuts have fruits with a lot of oil in them (also walnuts), but these are more or less exceptional cases. Their development is closely connected with the airy region through their many leaves. The strong tannin process which permeates the leaves indicates that the astral sphere is pulling at them strongly, for it controls and shapes air processes in the biological realm. These are no poisonous catkin bearers, for the astral nowhere overpowers their etheric or biological formative forces. One can see this in the insignificant or modest flowering process that lets the sprouting life of the shoots swing into it. This process tones the shooting life down but doesn't change it very much. It does not let it flame up, and it would not unleash its flowering power too soon and press it into showy petals. The germinal inflorescences are already there in the fall and most of them bloom in the spring. The Amentiflorae's shooting force creeps into its contracted catkins during the time when there is a general dampening of life. Then the flowering process is carried through the pure winter coolness with its crystalline clarity. It doesn't open and pour itself out passionately.

The basic plan for the amenti flowering plants is quite unified, but many varieties are possible. The solidifying earth element can generate hard oak and walnut woods or soft poplar woods. The watery element can participate to a greater or lesser extent. Their shapes can rise up in the air stiffly like poplar or they can blow into it like birches. We will now describe a few of the ones that have healing qualities.

Juglans regia – Common Walnut Tree

Walnut trees have nice shapes which reach out into the realm of light and air in a sturdy way, and they suck in light and warmth so intensely that other plants around them can only assert themselves with difficulty. A pungent smell wafts through the leafy, shadowy and bright crowns, each of the strongly ribbed, broad, pinnately compound leaves asserts itself in its space, and a somewhat egotistical health tolerates no beetles, worms, flies or ants. People think that one has to treat the trees roughly and that the nuts have to be beaten off with poles so that the trees will remain fertile. The wood in the often centuries old trunks with their light, smooth bark is heavy, dense, and hard.

The life at the ends of the annual shoots contracts into short, fat, female spikes, the long, green staminate catkin hang from the axils of last year's leaves, and after these two get through the winter they and the new leaves open up to the vernal winds around the beginning of May. Walnuts love brisk winds; they don't do well in damp, stuffy, valley air. The summer's heat lets the ovary swell into a green nut with a tight fitting, leathery but aromatically sharp, pungent husk, and a woody endocarp, the wrinkled cotyledons that are full of fat. Here cosmic warmth is condensed into oily substances. The whole formation has been separated out of the air into the region of earth forces and hard, solid and heavy things and when a noisy hail of nuts announces the walnut's harvest time it is a dramatic conclusion to the tree's year.

One gets a pungently aromatic, tasty tea from its boiled, young leaves; a decoction combats worms, parasites and vermin inside and out. Folk medicine uses leaf extracts as a bath and internally to treat scrofula, and tuberculous skins and mucous membranes.

One can understand the healing effects of Juglans regia if one observes how the tree places itself into air, light and warmth and draws them mightily towards it without dissolving or burning in them; it connects what it receives from the cosmos with its earthly solidity. The intensive tannin process in the leaf, husk and nutshell is an indication of the astral sphere that is working in the air, and the etheric oil and fatty oil point to the incorporation of the cosmic spheres of light and warmth. The fatty nut oil has a very unsaturated character and it becomes dense and tough on exposure to the air. That is why it is sometimes used as a drying agent in preparations of varnishes. Unsaturated fats are biologically valuable and active. Their relation to oxygen indicates that they are easily taken hold of by the etheric body and led over into live combustion processes where they become sources of warmth in the organism. Saturated fats tend to be deposited in the body.

However, the coarse, heavy nut with its hard shell and dense, solid wood show how earthy and earth bound our plant remains. In order to see how peculiar the whole walnut tree process is, just imagine a walnut tree that has the winged fruits of willow, poplars, birches or other catkin bearers.

Rudolf Steiner gave indications on how to obtain preparations from Juglans regia on two occasions. He suggested that one get tannic acid from the leaves and use it in the treatment of certain kinds of asthma and to alternate this with bitter substances from Veronica agrestis or other plants. There is an irregular activity of the astral body in asthma, especially in the bronchial, lung region. Also there is a "lack of appetite in the whole organism" which brings it about that foods are not taken into the circulation and rhythmic system in a healthy way. We cannot give more details here, but the function of tannins in connection with the activation of astral beings in plant life has been described in this work so often that we can refer the reader to the previous discussions.

Steiner's second indication was for the use of the nutshell. In a walnut one has "a real imitation of the astral body of a human being and one can use that in order to counteract deformations." Man's astral body is a totality, but it is differentiated in each organ region, so that each organ has its portion of the astral body's activity. Since the astral body mainly makes an impression in the gaseous organization of man's body (see the introductory section in Volume I), the astral body's activity in our breathing organ is especially important and interesting.

The nutshell, that contains a lot of tannins and its tannin process, with all of the astral connections which have been described so often, encloses the two leafy, plastic cotyledons that are swollen by the fat–forming process. The swelling forces which otherwise would make a juicy apple, for instance, are shriveled into a leathery, green husk. But they have not been lost. They have gone into the seed region and have made the cotyledons swell into something like a fruit. However, sap becomes oil in this region. Looked at from this viewpoint, an apple and a nut are contrasts. According to Rudolf Steiner, the thin–membraned core that houses the appleseeds, just as the membrane that encloses a nut, also imitates the part of the human astral body in its biological dynamics, but this time it is imitating the intestines instead of the lungs.

A look at our section on medicinal plants for the lungs will probably help the reader to understand this indication about walnut shells. There the lung is called an earth organ, and it is assigned to the solidification of the carbon process.

It should be mentioned that walnuts are hard nuts to crack. Healthy teeth will get a good workout when they crack them open.

Quercus robur – Red Oak

Calcium and Tannin

The oak shows us its strong, vital forces in its mighty, quiet growth into a giant tree, but it also makes a realm of counter forces visible in the dampening of these vital forces, so that the growth occurs slowly, ceaselessly but not stormily. The leaf that exhibits both expansion and contraction in its form tells us about the interaction of opposite forces. An acorn has both a plastic swelling and a scanty covering with a cup. After all the gnarled shape of the whole tree tells us about the battle with the tireless life that is constantly starting anew and being dampened again, and therefore does not simply shoot on in a straight line.

This oak vitality would proliferate in manifold ways if this dampening counter force was not incorporated in it. Oaks hand over their growth to strong mineralizing processes and let it be connected with earthy, heavy things, and they permit hard, heavy wood and thick bark to form. It takes about sixty to eighty years until the tree opens its first catkin and blossoms to the airy region, but the heavy fruit is quickly reclaimed by the earth as they fall to the ground. The flowering process is rather inconspicuous; no color or aroma makes it stand out from the leafy green of the crowns. However, a lot of animals show up around oaks, as if they would like to continue the etheric plant process into the astral sphere, as it were. No other tree harbors so many gall wasps and flies, each one of which stimulates a different kind of gall formation in the plant. This is stag beetle's territory, and blue jays sow the acorns with great artistry.

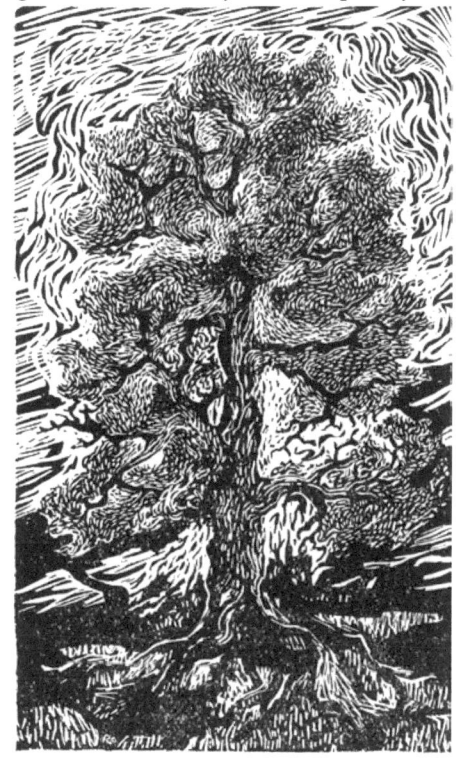

The oak's nature can be seen very clearly in the way it deals with two substances. It gets limestone out of the ground and permeates itself with calcium compounds in shoot, leaf, trunk and bark. One sometimes finds over 90% calcium oxide in the ashes of old bark. Rudolf Steiner pointed out that calcium is quite important in biological processes. It dampens etheric life forces when they would like to proliferate. It lets life contract in a healthy way, "without shock", and it gives the astral realms that are higher than etheric ones access to biological processes. Even in its mineral, metallic form, calcium has a strong connection with nitrogen, the substance in which the astral, soul element, incarnates. (We refer the reader to the section on legumes and Rubiaceae in Volume I of this work for an explanation of this statement. Also see the numerous other places that discuss nitrogen.) Calcium can burn directly in the nitrogen that otherwise smothers combustion. One can also see how strongly calcium attracts beings in the astral realm through the magnificent flowers on plants that grow in limestone.

The calcium process in the oak is complemented by an intensive tannin process. The latter is a plant organ for the reception of astral forces. It dampens proliferating life forces and brings formative forces into them, as one can see very nicely in oak leaves. One can also see the oak's proliferating power – although it is tamed – in the shapes of the acorns on the various species of oak (there are about 200 of them, and at least that many more have already died out). Threads, tongues, scales, soft thorns, and warts form on the outside of the cups, the proliferating forces want to break away everywhere, but they are restrained.

One of the oak's main organs is its bark, where its calcium and tannin processes meet each other in a particularly impressive way. The force with which an oak can throw itself into its bark formation can be seen in the cork oak, whose bark can be harvested every eight years right down to the trunk's parenchyma.

The large cupola on Rudolf Steiner's first Goetheanum was supported by seven pairs of columns that were made out of seven kinds of wood. The beech columns were followed by columns out of ash, cherry and oak. Then came columns out of elm, maple and birch. Each of the columns was an artistic representative of a different creative impulse in earth evolution and was assigned to a different planet, the two oak columns to Mars. The artistic language of the forms at the columns up to the oaken Mars column tells one something about the development of the earth out of spiritual elements until it became physically solid, and the Mercury, elm column and the following ones tell one about the earth's return to the spiritual. Earth evolution is divided into two halves. It descended from the spirit to the physical in a Mars–like way and has now begun to reascend from the physical into the spiritual in a Mercurial way. The oak condenses out of air and light into an iron hard tree with heavy fruits (it does best if one plants it in ascending Mars periods); it is really solidly at home in the earth. An oak forest tends to stay where it is; it doesn't spread out much. A little hill is an insurmountable barrier. The wood of an elm is also hard and solid, but it drops its light, winged fruits into the wind which bears them everywhere. The elm serves the winged and inspiring messenger Mercury, who shows one the way to one's heavenly home.

Remedies from oaks can help the I and astral body to shape and permeate the physical and to dampen the proliferating plastic, etheric principle that is active in all fluids, if it proves to be too strong. That is particularly important in childhood, when youngsters have to be led into their tasks on earth. The spirit must incarnate right down into the formation of bones. A basic remedy that was recommended by Rudolf Steiner for the regulation of children's calcium processes is a preparation out of oak bark and oyster shells, which contains a lot of calcium carbonate. This was supposed to be taken alternately with a preparation out of calcium phosphate and cucurbit flowers (see under "Gourds"). To understand this selection of substances one should realize that the formation of bark is not the result of anabolic processes but of dampened life that has been driven into the production and limiting of forms. Therefore it supports the influences that dampen life, gives form and proceed from the astral body and I which create man's consciousness and self–consciousness.

Another process in women which regulates their fertility rhythms after puberty and therewith serves the descent of souls into their bodies on earth, is also under the healing effect of the calcium process, which is an important component of blood activity; it carries formative processes into the blood and supports its ability to coagulate. Rudolf Steiner recommended the use of a basic remedy for the harmonization of human menstrual rhythms, which contains an oak bark preparation, plus shepherds purse, stinging nettle, marjoram and yarrow (Marjoram comp.).

Rudolf Steiner gave indications for another important oak bark preparation for the healing not of human beings but of sick soils and plants; this is one of the compost preparations used in biodynamic farming and gardening. A large number of the plant diseases which have increased in such an alarming way are due to agricultural methods that arose about 80 years ago and that are based on materialistic views. These methods have undermined plants' vitality and the health of topsoil, and have made cultivated plants subject to disease. The art of vitalizing the soil has been forgotten. The artificial fertilizers that are used so widely today stimulate the fluids in plants and drive them into a proliferating growth that cannot be permeated by formative forces and the plant's spiritual principle. The plant's constitution suffers, a foundation is created for the attack of parasites and an array of plant diseases spreads out. One tries in vain to gain control over the situation again with the strongest poisons (whose true nature one shamefully conceals under the name of "plant protecting agents"). The constitution of cultivated plants is weakened further. One has a mighty helper in the oak bark preparation if one wants to heal things from the ground up through the introduction of biodynamic agricultural methods. Like topsoil itself, oak bark is something that stands between living and dead things and between plant and mineral. The calcium in it that hasn't fallen completely out of the living realm yet is ideal for dampening proliferating life forces and thereby helping astral formative powers to control and organize these etheric forces. "One should use a calcium that has the structure of the kind that one finds in oak bark, so that this rampant etheric activity contracts in a regular and healthy way." (Rudolf Steiner)

Corylus Avellana – Filbert Shrub (European Hazelnut)

When hazelnut catkins stretch out and let their golden pollen drop into the early March winds, the earth is still moist and cool but the air is already dry and sunny. The very first prevernal life stirs, and bees dare to make their first flights to hazelnuts and snow drops. The tight buds pop, the hazelnut's essence breathes far out into the illumined atmosphere and the thawed watery element rises into the air. However, just as a cloud contracts again into a fructifying shower of drops after it has absorbed enough cosmic forces, so a fructifying cloud of pollen sinks down upon the feathery purple stigmas of the "female" flowers and brings the light, warmth, dryness, solar and astral quality of the sphere it goes through to the receptive drop on the stigma, which has risen like springing life from the moist depths of the earth.

Looked at from the musical perspective, the sixth, seventh and octave sounds of blooming and fertilizing that have sounded so early dim down, and the fruits' further development is hidden and quiet for many weeks and months. The aments fall off, the naked bush stands in its prime tone, until late—in April in its querying second and weaving third—the leafy hands that are all inclined towards the dark earth open, are slowly lifted up by the light, and they then spread out joyfully and wide while the new shoots ascend like trumpet blasts. Life becomes consolidated as in the fourth, the leaves become coarser, shooting life reaches its limits for the year. The summery growth fifth sounds and the inner and outer elements' boundaries touch each other.

Even though the strong, vital forces of a hazelnut can be seen in its rapid growth and in its tough, indestructible ability to send up new shoots from every stump, its wood is solid and elastic. Its broad leaves are snugly attached to the new shoots, they have no long stems and they don't divide or form feathers. The shrub now lives entirely in its leafy greenness, for the slowly developing fruits are hidden in enveloping, leafy husks. A hazelnut remains connected with the light and warmth sphere at this stage of its development; it gathers solar forces through its leaves during the whole summer and fall, and it streams them towards its ripening nuts that are slowly closing themselves off with a woody shell. A nut's mild, dry oil that is as sweet as almonds is warmth that has become substance. The warmth cosmos has become fruitful in the heavy earthly realm.

From the way the leaf buds and the developing leaves point downwards one can see why people used to make divining rods out of hazelnut branches. On the other hand, the whole, vital plant lifts itself so resolutely into the air, light and warmth that one also sees why clairvoyants used to sense the friendly, beneficial nature of this bush and why they liked to find it and plant it in thickets, at the edge of woods, along brooks and elsewhere. They considered it to be a snake repellent, and bountiful harvests of nuts indicated that all living creatures in the area were going to be fruitful. Their experience of the harmonious light and fire power in the hazelnut process that connected it with chthonic earth powers could become Imaginations like the following: the earth mother with its heavenly child resting well hidden under the bush that is never touched by the lightning that is flashing all around it.

Hazel bushes were planted around the Goetheanum in Dornach, that center of modern spiritual science, a protective wall against the anti-spiritual forces that would like to cut off the earth and man from the spiritual cosmos and from the being who created the world. (Also quince trees, to provide counter forces against the power of false spiritualization, which would like to flee the places where earthly tasks are done, out of an egotistical longing for heaven.)

WILLOWS – SALICACEAE

Salicin and Tannin Processes

Whereas the catkin bearers that we have gotten to know so far have been plants in which the illumined airy element is connected with the solid, earthy elements (walnut, oak, hazelnut), the willows are plants where the airy element permeates that which is cool and moist. We have a relatively young plant family before us, which appeared in the Tertiary Period for the first time, but only really developed at the end of the Atlantean period of earth evolution, or after the Ice Age. The Atlantean, foggy atmosphere became cleansed from the watery element during those mighty catastrophes that mankind has remembered in its flood sagas: the air now had some warmth and light from the sun passing through it. (See Rudolf Steiner's *Occult Science* and *Cosmic Memory*). The glaciers melted, glacial seas and moors arose and the great hour of the willows and birches struck, the hour of the trees that always congregate in light filled groves and never in dense forests.

Thus cool and moist things belong to willows, and so do illumined growing places. They populate the northern temperate zone, high up into glacial and polar meadows. They follow the banks of brooks, grow along the edges of woods and moors, they fill the river meadows and damp, low spots with the willow thickets which European botanists know as salicidoms. They love flowing or bubbling water and illumined air. Willow shoots grow rapidly out of the damp, fresh ground that gives their roots plenty of water, and they show their exuberant vitality in their ability to grow roots from any twig that is cut off.

These strong, vital forces don't like to be restricted to rigid forms. A fluctuating and variable tendency runs through the whole family. Their leaf forms range from pussy willow's roundish ovals to the finely serrated, lanceolate leaves of white willows. The leaf forms tell one whether the rounding formative forces are more active or less so. Willow species are not firmly fixed, because they are constantly cross–pollinating, to the despair of the classifiers who find it difficult to distinguish and determine things here. Sometimes the leaves act like flowers and have their own nectarine; this shows that they are touched by the higher regions which only belong completely to flowers. The flower buds open at the beginning of spring; the airy, wind-blown catkins slip out of their shimmering, silky hairs and become the "palm" branches of Easter time.

Shortly thereafter, at the end of spring, the feathered willow seeds with fuzzy tufts of hair separate from the twigs, float away with every puff of the wind, and for a short time they belong entirely to the illumined airy element that was formatively active on the willow right from the time its life began. Willows also love the airy element in water; their roots look for oxygenated water many meters down in the ground and can run into defective, porous water or waste conduits which they then plug up by growing side roots. Willows don't keep the water they suck up, they exhale most of it into the atmosphere and thus weave water into the airy element.

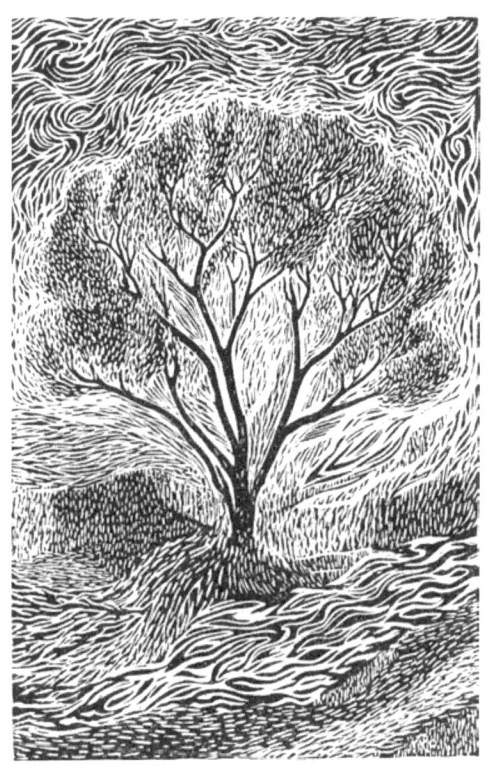

The many flexible branches which spring so easily from willows – the gift and harvest of this plant is its branches – show the water how to pass into the air. They remain flexible because they preserve an unhardened plastic life, and they keep their insides fluid, which is something that basket weavers are looking for. It also makes it easy for the wind to blow them around. If one looks at a white willow that is rooted in a river bank on a windy, sunny day, it is very easy to see how its roots are assigned to streaming water and its shimmering leaf region to moving air and flowing light. Thus the willow process stands at the boundary between two realms of nature, and it leads water out of its realm and into the blowing wind.

However, a willow has a close connection with a realm that is influenced and shaped by its particular nature, and not just with the air. It is plant life existence presses towards the astral world which weaves in air and ensouls the animals that flit around in it. The blooming catkins attract bees and offer them a vernal repast. They and the butterflies, beetles, two and four–winged flies smell the fine, sweet and dry fragrance and they bear the pollen through the air. Many beetles, gall wasps, flies and worms live in willows, and birds nest in them. Here again one sees that the willow process is trying to unite strong vital forces with the higher (astral) forces that are raying in from the animals.

The transition of water into the airy which willows are involved in a great deal, means as much for earthly life as the transition of plant life into animal existence does, namely, it opens up lower forces to a higher condition.

The willow process also expresses itself in a characteristic way in the substances it produces, such as tannins and salicylic compounds. The latter are named after willows (salix), since they were first discovered in the bark.

We don't have to go into the nature of the tannin process here since we have done this from various viewpoints already. It will suffice to remind ourselves that the tannin-filled bark of a tree is an organ that attracts the cosmic, astral forces which must envelop the plant's shoots and leaves so that its etheric body receives impulses that let the higher flowering nature proceed from the leaf process. It is not easy for really vigorous plants that have connected themselves strongly with the watery element that is the bearer of plastic, etheric, formative forces to let the astral element work into them. The latter is always connected with the airy element that wants to assert itself, and it has to dampen life processes and the watery element. For instance, water lilies, mangroves (that live in tropical swamps near the coast) and tormentils provide a lot of tannins.

Tannins that combine with sugar are present in plants as glycosides. They course through the plant's fluidic system and they like to collect in the bark and trunk, older leaves, fruits and other parts that are becoming dry and solid. They never circulate in aromatic substances or ones that are evaporating into the air.

The formation of salicylic compounds is a second characteristic activity of willows and it is related to such volatilization. Salicylic compounds are found in plants that raise themselves particularly intensively out of the watery, etheric realm into airy, fragrant flowering activity, as in willows, pansies, primulas, swamp birches, meadowsweets and wintergreens. Thus salicylic acid and its compounds also have to do with the permeation of the etheric with the astral.

Salicylic acid is found in willows in various forms. Connected with sugar as a glycoside, it is a water soluble substance that circulates in plants and deposits near the bark. This gives it a certain connection with tannins. However, near the flower region the salicylic process changes, sheds its sugar and connects itself with certain alcohols. Now we have a substance that is like essential oils and flower fragrances—something volatile which belongs in the airy region. Here the salicylic process becomes raised into a region that remains inaccessible to the tannin process.

The material properties of salicylic acid prepare it for such a transition. It is water soluble and it evaporates with the water if one boils the solution. Salicylic acid goes up into the region where plants flower and become fragrant, whereas tannins move towards rigidifying, solid forms, they deposit in barks and woods and they tan proteins and keep them from rotting. The common feature in plants that develop a lot of salicylic acid is that a rampant, watery element tears itself away from the watery region and passes into an airy, flowering one.

Willow bark has long been used as a remedy in the treatment of feverish colds, especially the rheumatic kind. Rudolf Steiner recommended a preparation of ferns and willow leaves for the regulation of the digestive processes and to aid the rhythmic processes of the whole gastro–intestinal tract. Here willow forces have a mediating effect between various regions, just as they do in the nature processes described above. The curative effect of willow bark on chronic diarrhea is such that the siphoning off of liquids from the intestines returns to normal. The appetite is stimulated, that is, the whole organisms sympathy for the nutritional process is enhanced. The bark's diaphoretic effect in colds points to a warming and a control of the fluidic system, which surrendered itself too strongly to the cold and gravity of the outer world and became bogged down, as it were. Its effects on the lungs, skin and rheumatic joints are connected with boundary surfaces where a fluidic process is being regulated. Thus fluidic processes are everywhere subjected to the effects of the astral body; the latter receives a push to give more intense impulses for a proper warming and aeration of our fluidic system after it has withdrawn from this activity for a while. If one takes mineralized willow bark instead of the leaves, the I that is engaged in the fine mineralization activities is drawn into the process. The astral body becomes receptive for the I's activity.

Betula pendula – European White Birch

Among the many beautiful kinds of catkin trees, one has to crown the noble birch; that is a queen's crown, for we attribute womanly loveliness to a birch. It is the eternally girlish, young princess of bright, northern groves and woods. It is married to the light and wind, it dissolves its whole form in the illumined air, and even the trunk that is "protruding earth" is like a column of light. The silvery white veneer that covers the dark bark is unique. Where could a light green May be more beautiful than in a birch arbor, and what could celebrate a spiritually illumined Whitsun festival more worthily than birch leaves on their branches in Maytide? Even the darkness of a moor that is populated by melancholic or spooky junipers and heather is dispelled if a luciferous birch with its salutary fragrance takes root there. Birke, bircha, biricha or bjork in ancient and Nordic languages may be connected with Berchta the magnificent and bright, and it would then mean the shimmering or resplendent one.

And in fact the sounds in the word "Birke" express what an eye that feels the world experience in a birch; the light vowel I that is connected with R the movement sound is consolidated in K and lovingly embraced by B. Eurythmy, the new art of movement that is "visible speech" can make the speech form of such a word visible and it makes one aware that our tree was given a name that describes its real nature. The birch is the eurythmist among trees and it lets the wind that sighs through it take on forms and come to visible speech through a continual shaping process with blowing veils and a streaming flow of movement. Air strives towards its highest form in speech. Our tree loves the lands of the "Hyperborean Apollo" with its rhythmic alternation of cool, strict formative power and long hours of light, and it is not so keen about the southern regions with its rampant life and incubating warmth. It prefers granite soils and the primal rocks that contain silica—the light substance. Shrub birches conquer the arctic regions and high mountains. A birch sucks in the cool waters in brooks from mountains and glaciers and in moors, and it exhales the fluidic element into the air so that it is like a remedy for waterlogged soils. One can see right away that bark is one of the birch's main organs. Its bark takes in many forces which other trees give to their twigs and leaves, flowers and fruits. In spite of the silvery white outer skin, birch bark soon becomes dark and hard as iron, in contrast to the soft, light wood. It proves to be almost indestructible and impervious to water, and many people in the north find that it is a good material for making roofs, boxes, scabbards and canoes. The bark contains aromatic, camphorous materials (such as betuline) like those in flowers, and nutrients that can supplement one's diet in times of need. Betula lenta (blackberry birch) even has sugar in its bark.

Birches excrete a lot of things into their bark which would otherwise develop in flowers' color and aroma and in the weight and sweetness of fruits. The tree remains unfinished and forever young at the top; it doesn't consolidate itself in the formation of a strong crown (as Gerbert Grohmann pointed out). Rudolf Steiner was the first one to draw our attention to the most important part of this strange separation process. He pointed out that birches differ from all other plants in that they separate two processes in their roots and elsewhere that otherwise merge; salt absorption and the formation of proteins. Birch sap contains a lot of potassium salts and they wind up in the bark, and the proteins that thereby become salt free go 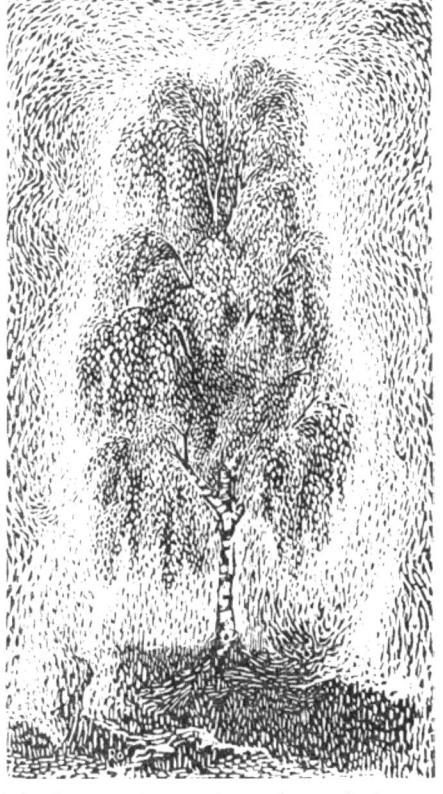 into the leaves. So the branches' bark contains an intensive salt (especially potassium) process, and birch leaves have a special protein process that is freed from salty things. If these two processes had been united from the roots on, one would get a "wonderful blooming and fruit bearing herb" (R. Steiner), and not a birch form.

This peculiarity gives birches their special healing qualities. The leaves and their salt free protein process and the bark and their intensive salt process can work upon quite different regions in the human organization. To understand this twofold healing tendency of birches, one has to know about the two poles that are present in man's organization. They were described by Rudolf Steiner in Lecture 15 of his cycle *Spiritual Science and Medicine* that was given to doctors around Easter in 1920. Anabolic protein processes and processes that form and excrete salts are present in birches and human bodies. But the formations of proteins and salts are connected with different organs, members of man's being and regions in the overall human being. One can look at a "central man" who is concentrated in the metabolic organs of the "lower organization." In the transformation and building up of human protein one is confronted by a "peripheral man" who is active from the upper, nerve–sense pole primarily located in the head. The latter is engaged in breakdown activities and salt formation, and mineralizes the living protein that is created by the "central man", in a very fine way. One could say that the "central man" tends more towards the animal side, since the physical, etheric and astral bodies that constitute the animal mainly work together in it, whereas there is a tendency in the "peripheral man" to withdraw and free the spiritual members, to leave them to themselves and to only let their imprints work in the body. Thereby one's spirit can arrive at consciousness and self-consciousness, while the physical tends to become mineralized.

One's spiritual I and highest member must keep control over all these processes. Otherwise one gets pathological processes or aberrations towards the animal side or the mineral one. "If you take leaves which conserve forces that form protein, you get that part of the birch which especially goes toward the central man and which will prove to be a good remedy for gout and rheumatism." (R. Steiner) The favorable effects of a salt free diet on the various diseases that are connected with deposits and hardening became manifest recently in the so-called Gerson diet. However, one has a unique salt free protein in birch leaves that arose in a natural way. Birch bark works more upon the "peripheral man". If the latter and the processes that are peculiar to its nature does not interact with the processes that proceed from the "central man" in the right way (the interaction of both poles constitutes the whole person) one gets congestions and deposits of uncontrolled, hardened, mineralized, breakdown materials. Things must become "de-salted", and birch bark preparations are helpful here.

From about age 35 on, there is danger because the catabolic tendencies of the "upper peripheral" pole of the body begin to predominate over the anabolic ones of the "lower, central" man. The latter's activities can be suitably reinforced through cures with birch leaf preparations at regular intervals, say in the spring, so that it can stand up to the attacks of the "peripheral man" that now occur to a greater extent. Rudolf Steiner recommended such rejuvenation cures to all those who are over 35.

The birch is a tree that remains youthful to a high degree and it helps to unite youthfulness and a healthy aging. For the "central man" is supposed to preserve youthfulness, and the "peripheral man" to bring in the maturing forces of later years. If these two are united in the right way, the health that is appropriate for the second half of life is maintained.

Rues – Rutaceae
Masters of Tropical Warmth Processes

In Volume I of this work we tried to describe the nature of plant families like the labiata that permit themselves to be permeated and shaped by cosmic warmth processes to an extraordinary extent. These influences induce such plants to produce essential oils, which are special warmth substances. If the formative warmth processes go into the trunk and roots or solidifying region one gets aromatic balsams and resins.

Such "warmth substances" will work curatively upon man's warmth system and upon the spiritual I that is particularly active in the latter.

This cosmic action of warmth varies, depending on the way that it is accompanied by many kinds of earthly processes, spatially and temporally. Vernal warmth is different from summery and autumnal warmth. The warmth of our northern temperate zone is different from tropical heat or that warmth of the southern temperate zone. The sun that rays down to us during the course of the year has twelve different effects. The sun in Cancer has a different effect than in Libra or Sagittarius. A Piscean sun is connected with vernal processes on our part of the earth, with summery events in the tropics and with autumnal ones in Argentina and New

Zealand. Warmth retains more of its cosmic purity near the poles, and it becomes earthy in the tropics. Head warmth is different from heart warmth or liver warmth, and we have to evaluate the warmth of a Norwegian summer day differently than Sicilian, Indian or Australian warmth during the time when the sun is shining out of Gemini, high for us and low for the southern hemisphere.

Thus the cosmic formative process for essential oils is opposed by various factors, depending on the earth process with which it connects itself. The earth exhales a copy of this differentiating warmth activity in the scents and fragrances of its plants. One could say that each aroma is like a spectral line in the warmth spectrum.

The warmth processes that are organized in rues are mainly tropical ones, for most of their 900 plus species live near the equator. Only a few venturesome ones come up into our regions. In the tropics the type mainly forms trees with hard and often resinous woods, bitter or aromatic barks, coarse, evergreen and very aromatic leaves that mostly have smooth edges and are dotted with etheric, transparent oil glands, and an extensive flowering process. The flowers are symmetrical stars that are often white, their aromas are sweet and voluptuous, desire and fulfillment at the same time. Evanescent charm wafts towards us from lemon blossoms, a sweet fullness from orange blossoms, a somewhat tart invigoration from the leaves of citrus plants and a pleasantly refreshing tang from the rinds of their fruit. The perfume of cologne is mainly based on a mixture of the scents of the leaves, flowers and fruits of these and related "warmth plants."

The type becomes a hard-leafed shrub in the subtropics and on jungle mountains, and an herb in the temperate zones. Rue and fraxinella are the last scouts that reach our climes; they flee the cold zones further north.

There is a large variety of Rutaceae fruits. The tropics furnish us with sour, sweet juicy fruits like grapefruit, oranges, lemons, tangerines and mangos but also with fiery, peppery berries. The watery and earthly elements press up powerfully into the warm region around juicy fruits. The latter sometimes form leathery, wooden shells, or they lignify completely. The shells often split and release winged fruits. Some of the tropical Rutaceae are small, thorny trees; they oppose tropical swelling and proliferating forces with their strict formative forces; they are well formed plants. A salutary, refreshing process against the incubating monotonous tropical sultriness and the wet tropical heat is prepared in the sour–sweet fruit sap and in the invigorating aroma. The general tendency of the Rutaceas' healing effects will be in the direction of an interaction between the warmth and fluidic organisms; they will combat a chaotic proliferation and swelling of the lower organization against the upper one, dampen the "tropical" regions of the warmth system and the centrifugal inflammatory and loosening processes, and they will strengthen the formative forces of the I and astral body that are active in the air and warmth organization. We will give more details about this in our discussion of four medicinal plants in this family, after we make a survey of the various species into which the type is distributed over the earth.

South Africa with its dry steppes and desert has 180 Diosma species, which are small shrubs with simple leathery leaves and very fragrant flowers. Tropical Australia has 180 Boronioceas, which are shrubs with small, simple leaves and leathery glands and beautiful flowers. Agathosma is a group of small, thorny trees with yellow wood and of very fragrant bushes in the rocky steppes on the Mexican mountains. There are 140 species of Fagora in the West Indies, and 100 Cusparoideas in tropical America, which are hardwood trees or thorny fragrant shrubs that contain a lot of resin. However, the Aurantoidea with their spicy leaves and juicy fruits are the biggest group in the family, and they grow in the hot sections of Asia.

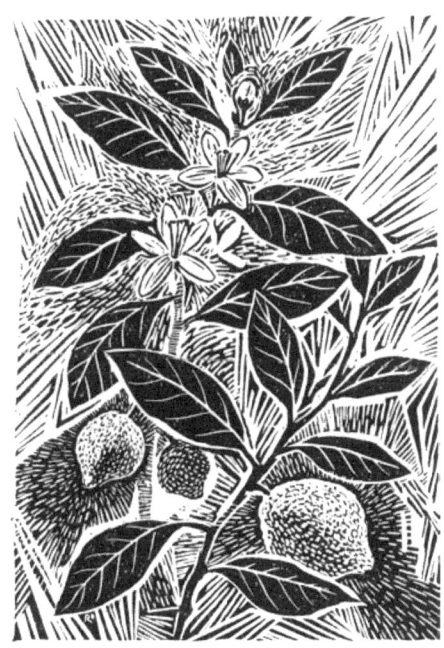

Citrus limonum – Lemon Tree

The formative forces of south and southeast Asia produced the original lemons, oranges, tangerines and their relatives. The forests on the south sides of the mountains near India and China still include the wild form of the lemon tree, a tough, thorny plant with hard wood.

The one pole of this sphere

of formative forces is characterized by a mighty sucking up of rampant earth forces and a swelling up and rising up of the absorbed, enlivened water to exuberant tropical life, and the other pole shows up as an intensive inhalation and "earthifying" of the cosmic light and warmth forces. In this tropical growth earth processes are taken in and streamed outwards in a centrifugal manner, whereas cosmic processes are sucked into the leaves and become manifest as a tendency towards volatilization and atomization in the heavy tropical aromas and the luxurious scents of the flowers, or they load up the leaves, barks, woods and fruits with thousands of spicy substances.

Each lemon tree interacts with these rampant life forces and lets them endow it with as many as 2000 lemons in one year, and yet it tones down and controls this exuberance. A small tree stands before us, broadly rooted and branched and decorated with dense, evergreen foliage. The flowering process takes hold of it in a big way with many reddish white blossoms that envelop it in a cloud of sweet, evanescent and intoxicating aromas, which tells one about the intensive permeation of its etheric formative forces organization with an (astral) spherical sheath that intensifies its life beyond itself towards an almost animal existence, although the plant is unable to incorporate this spherical sheath, for only an animal organization can do this. The intervention is so strong that the leaves form scents like those in flowers, although they are duller and not as perfect, whereas its flowers intensify this process to the utmost and translate the centrifugal unfolding tendencies with a release of sweetly fragrant waves of scent into its environment.

An energetic formation of fruits immediately counters this dissipation. The sap in the swelling ovary that is pressing outwards becomes enclosed by a firm, leathery shell so that the tropical heat cannot cook or sweeten it very much. The intensive formation of acids that is peculiar to unripe fruits is sustained, and only a little sugar is formed. Acids are usually oxidized when fruits ripen, but in this case they are kept at an unripe stage for a long time. In lemons sugar formation is suppressed in favor of acid formation. The sugar process is directed towards the formation of the strongest, tricarboxylic fruit acid (citric acid)[10] and towards the formation of the related ascorbic acid or vitamin C. The aro-

---

[10] See the formula for this below in the section on the Oxolidaceae

matization process that is peculiar to our plant and is present in its leaves and flowers, is changed again in the rind; it is now refreshing and stimulating, rather than dull and smoldering as in the leaf, or sweet and intoxicating as in the flower.

Thus a lemon is a particularly characteristic formation on a lemon tree. Limiting, enclosing centripetal, formative tendencies begin to counteract the previously described centrifugal tendencies in fruit formation. Citrus fruits stand between two contrasts in the fruit formation that we encounter in plants. One can see that the watery element predominates in juicy berries, whereas in dry, woody capsules there is a suppression and expulsion of fluids and of the etheric forces that induce swellings; a lemon is in between these two poles. It permits fluids to well up as in a berry, but it encloses them with a leathery, half hardened rind that is permeated by the formative forces of airy and warmth elements. (In close relatives of the lemon such as the balsamocitrus tree, the fruit rind becomes hard wood that encloses sweet, aromatic orange flesh.)

If one cuts through a lemon one can distinguish four zones. They make the four formative forces in a plant's etheric body manifest in a way that is characteristic for lemons. One sees the action of warmth ether in the volatile, combustible, essential oils in the outer yellow rind that are born from warmth. One also sees the action of light ether in the bright color that comes from the carotenes that assimilate light in the dynamics of the plant. In human and animal organisms carotenes become the Vitamin A which protects all organs that develop from the ectoderm from drying and dying processes, and which is concentrated in the visual purple that is present in our eyes. These carotenes are related to citrate, and the latter is the base for lemon peels' aroma.

The yellow layer encloses a white one which is spongy and airy; it contains pectins and bitter substances and one can see that it has been made by light and air. Then comes the widest zone, that is full of juice; firmly encircled by the first two layers, it is assigned to the watery element and the living, chemical formative forces that become manifest in Vitamin C and other fruit acids, sugars, mucilages, gums and minerals that fill the juice. The mineral substances in the juice that are raised into the living realm include calcium, potassium, a little silicic acid and a trace of boron. The latter is generally present in nectars, fruits and plant parts that contain sugar, and it is connected with the centrifugal process that puts the sugar that is formed in the leaves out into the flower and fruit region.

The fourth region near the center of the fruit belongs to solids and the life ether. It contains numerous very vital seeds that germinate easily and that are covered by a slimy, bitter layer; however, this slime strongly inhibits germination. Taking a brief look at lemon juice we see that it contains about 7–7.5% citric acid, 0.5% malic acid, 2.5% sugar, 0.4% pectins and glucides and 0.2% ashes with the mineral ingredients given above. The acid content fluctuates, depending on what time of the year the lemons were harvested, for the trees produce them practically all year round. This content is greatest in fruits that are harvested in November: this is the time when life contracts and gets weaker and when centrifugal forces weaken. When the latter get stronger again in the spring in connection with the earth's whole life, the juice's acid content decreases.

Thus the salutary totality that we have before us in lemon juice is composed of manifold acids that are still connected with the carbohydrate process of the formation of aromatic and bitter substances like those that are more prevalent in the rind, and of calcium potassium and other minerals that have been raised to plant level. (Investigators have recently become more interested in the significance of the citric acid cycle in man's metabolism.) These material events draw one's attention to the processes that stand behind them and produce them. The dissolving, centrifugal processes in the tropics are the opposite of these processes, and the latter enable one to understand the tonic effect of lemon juice, which holds man's members together in a centripetal way. The things that try to move out centrifugally into a formless state are pressed back and tamed. The breakdown and shaping tendencies that mainly become active through man's upper organization are strengthened against the lower, vegetative, metabolic system, or the warmest, "tropical" organ region that we have in us. Rudolf Steiner was the first to recommend lemon juice preparations for hay fever, and we can now see why they can be effective (e.g. Gencydo). Citrus medications are also indicated for colds, rheumatic diseases, dropsy and prescorbutic conditions in the spring. In short, they can be used for all conditions in which the fluidic system threatens to become formless and out of control and where one has to come to the assistance of the shaping and tissue toning activities of the upper organization that should be in control of things, and where centripetal formative tendencies should be strengthened against the centrifugal tendencies that have taken over.

Ruta graveolens – Rue

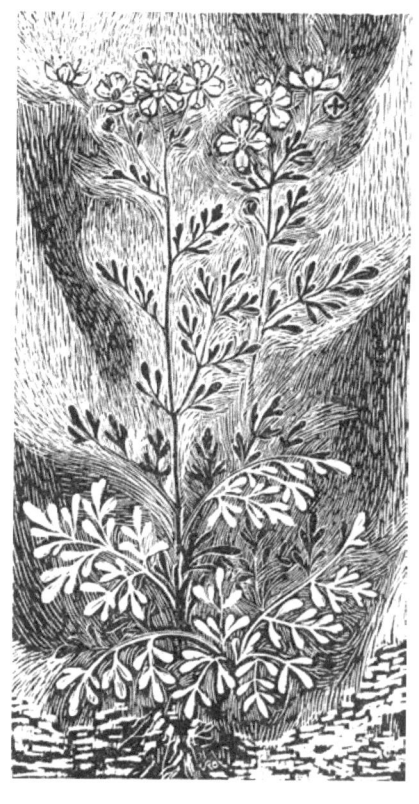

The Rutacea type sends its last stragglers into the Mediterranean region. Rue has become an herb there that lignifies down below, and it grows on hot, rocky limestone soils. It was probably grape growers who brought it over the Alps and monks cultivated them in their gardens and some of them escaped and took root in suitably warm places elsewhere. The yellow and green herb proliferates, and the forms of its leaves show that a plastic, rounding tendency is battling one that wants to make pinnate forms. The shoots have many leaves, and in June its inflorescence opens up into cymes of flat, four petaled yellow and green flowers. A dully spicy scent permeates the whole plant that smells something like tangerine peels, although the smell is duller and slightly acid, like smoke from wet wood. Handling the leaves can produce inflammations, swelling, blisters and similar injuries. One can see that too many fire and light forces are working down into the swelling, fluid region that carry the flowering and fruiting impulse into the leafy region. The warmth element can be seen in the formation of essential oils and the light element in the creation of rutin and other yellow dyes. The fruits are dried out capsules.

This warmth plant with its strong flowering process that extends right into the leaves has an effect on man's blood organ that thereby becomes more active with regard to his lower organization. As the blood rushes in there, metabolic activity becomes intensified, hindrances to menstruation are overcome and muscles are strengthened. The I is urged to become more active in the metabolism. The voluntary use of eye and other muscles is facilitated. We know that the will's action is inhibited in sluggish metabolic processes. If the I organization and astral body are held up at the surface of an organ so that they don't permeate and organize it, one can get cramps; Rudolf Steiner said that this was the cause of epileptic seizures. Rue is one of many medicinal plants that were once used for this kind of problem, but Steiner recommended plants like Belladonna and Hyoscyamus instead (for epilepsy). The old herbalists used to say that rue was an antidote for poisons and that it made people more resistant to contagious diseases. As we often mentioned, abnormal astral forces are at work in plant poisons. However rue elaborates these astral forces, and it is not a very poisonous plant. In its formation of essential oils it devotes itself to cosmic warmth processes that have an egoistic nature. (See what was said about labiata in Volume I). Plants that form a lot of essential oils are generally not poisonous plants; the cosmic I impulses remain the master of the astral influences in them. If the human I impulse is strong enough, it is a powerful help against contagious diseases and other influences from outside. As we said about Angelica (see vol. 1), rue was considered to be a plant that wards off pestilences.

It is not too surprising that this plant has an effect on our light organ or eye, since it elaborates the light process in it so intensively that it produces a lot of yellow dye, rutin.

Dictamnus albus – Burning Bush – Fraxinella – Gas Plant

Growing up to three feet high this plant is another Rutacea at the northern end of the type's geographical range. Its whitish branded rhizome sends up shoots with pinnately compound, shiny, firm leaves in the spring, that go over into luxuriant, pyramidal clusters of flower buds at their tips. These open in June into flat flowers that are similar in form and color to horse-chestnut blossoms, although the petals are more pointed, whitish red, with a strong and sultry smell, like lemons and cinnamon. The five–pointed flower form is deformed by gravity, four petals rise from their base and the lowest one hangs down; the stamens and styles bend upwards at first or extend far out from their base, but they sink after awhile. The fruit is a hard capsule after it matures and dries, which then pops open and hurls its black seeds with a choleric gesture.

An inner fire process permeates this plant that likes dry, calcareous, sunny spots such as vineyard slopes, rocky hill- sides and dry meadows. Its stem, leaves and fruits are dotted with glands full of etheric oil, and a strong lemon smell mixed with one like caraway seeds, that is dull and refreshing, clings to the hand that rubs over it. This is really a "hot" plant that stands in its own aura of warm gases and it exhales an inflammable vapor.

Its healing effects are similar to those of rue, it fires up metabolic processes, brings on menstruation and eases gynecological ailments. This plant was also used as an anti-epileptic. In the Middle Ages it was advocated as an antidote for poisons and to ward off contagious illnesses.

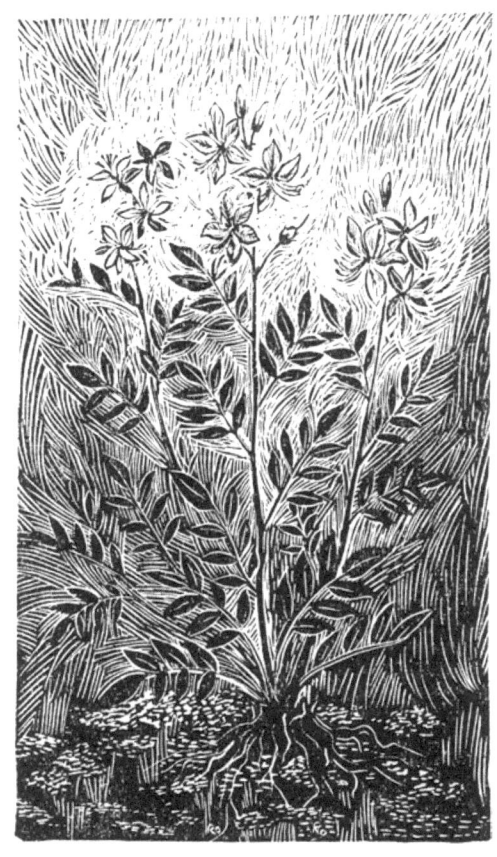

Barosma betulinum – Buchu

The Rutaceae family also sends a few species down to the southern tip of Africa, besides the ones it sends north to Mediterranean climes. The man–high Buchu shrub with leaves like those on birches is a real Ruta plant with its opposite, small, glossy green, strongly aromatic leaves dotted with glands containing etheric oil that crowd around the stem and branches, and with its white flowers in the axils with a heavy, sweet smell. The fruit is a five-celled capsule.

The leaves of Buchu have a strongly aromatic taste and an odor that is partly like peppermint and partly like rosemary, and a tea or an extract prepared from them has a warming, stimulating effect on the region around the kidneys, bladder and sexual organs, and combats chronic inflammations there.

Pinks – Caryophyllaceae

Chickweeds, Stitchworts, Campions

The Pink family type seems to have decided to make the stem its main organ and therewith to mainly live in straight lines. This stem is erected in species with large, showy flowers like clove pink, coat flower, feathered pink, sweet William, corncockle, campions, cockscomb, bitter root, Four o'clock and Bouncing Bet. It develops more branches in the gypsophilas, where a larger number of blossoms compensates for their smaller size. In the chickweeds and pearl weeds the stem begins to creep and to branch out in mats as in starweeds, tongue grass, spurry, nailwort, pearlwort, purslane, herniary and baby's breath. Here the flowers become small and humble, and they lose in colors and scents while they gain in tough vitality, and become weeds and plants on beaches, steppes and high mountains. However, the mountain types begin to develop more beautiful albeit delicate flowers through the cosmic influences in the heights. Every European mountain climber has seen mountain pinks, Alpine campions, etc.

The narrow, undivided, grasslike leaves that often shoot out of the nodes without petioles also seem to be formed out of the stem's linear element. They can become fine as needles, draw close to the stem as scabs, or get a little wider in species that like shady, moist places. Their similarity to the grasses is great, since they also shoot up in long stems, branch out and form mats, cushions and tufts.

Nodes and pairs of leaves proceed rhythmically up the stem in such growth, and the uniform repetition does not at first permit any metamorphosis or change of the basic motif into more elaborate formations. One has to look upon this strongly rhythmical element and this intensive development of stem and leaves as an essential feature in a pink. It remains at the herb level and doesn't get into tree formation.

After this rhythmical process along the stem has warded off the metamorphic intervention of a higher formative principle long enough; the plant does finally go over into an intensive flowering process that makes pinks into blooming flowers that consume life forces into flowery fire. This is a strong contrast to the grasses, whose flowering process remains modest and doesn't ignite even though it connects itself with the airy element. Gerbert Grohmann, the pioneer of a botany that has been extended by spiritual science, pointed out that this renunciation enabled grasses to become food and bread plants; however pinks cannot do this. There are a lot of ornamental plants among them and also some medicinal 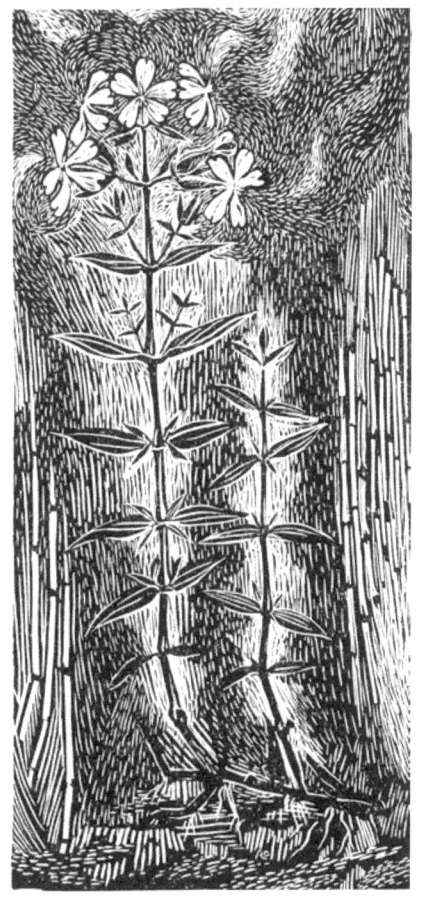 plants. Many of them are slightly toxic due to the delayed flowering process, which then breaks in quite strongly; nevertheless they would poison any bread that one would make out of their seeds. That's why corn cockle seeds must be carefully separated from grain when it is threshed so that they don't get into the flour and bread.

This points to an important process that is connected with the way that the astral realm and its beings interact with the pink's etheric principle, which results in the formation of toxins. The intensive flowering process points to a strong penetrating of the astral realm; but the latter is received by a well developed rhythmic system, so that only a moderate amount of toxins is formed. Here one gets saponins instead of alkaloids. Since we have often described the nature of the saponin process in this

Healing Plants (see the indices and especially the section on Primulaceae below), it will suffice to mention that Caryophyllaceae are one of the saponin containing families in the plant kingdom.

Corncockle, soap wort and rupture wort are familiar traditional medicinal plants in the family.

This family with its roughly 1800 species is at home in rhythmic climes, [11]especially in the northern temperate zone; it presses up mountain sides and into cold regions, but it stays away from the tropics. It likes light, open and dry spaces rather than wet ones, such an environment suits its formative nature the best. The happy, even passionate, flowers often have long tubes, their sepals sometimes tend to dry out, and some of the latter are like flaming feathers with the active colors of the spectrum, white, yellow and red. The blown up calyces, in soapwort, campions and others express a tendency to take hold of the airy element, which is one side of the saponin process. Some aspects of pinks remind one of the primrose family, but the latter belong to the spring and the former to summer; pinks are more fiery.

If one uses what is said about saponins in the section on Primulaceae as a guideline, one will see how medicinal pinks can stimulate the human organism. Then one will understand why one can use latherwort and rupture wort as diuretics, expectorants and a harmonizer of the blood and breathing organs.

Rudolf Steiner once recommended a preparation of the resin of Lychnis viscaria (catch fly, Pitch Pink) as an adjuvant treatment for pulmonary consumption in a senior citizen. In order to see why he did so one will probably have to look at the carbon process that is condensed in the intensive stem formation on the one hand, and at the condensed "sulfuric" process in the formation of resins and balsams in this stem on the other. Resins and pitches generally occur at the upper end of each stem. One can find the whole three-membered plant in this section of the stem; the node from which it springs is like a root that is based on the plant below it, the middle pieces reflects the rhythmic region, and at the upper end the stem contracts again in anticipation of the flower formation. It is precisely in this upper part that "pitch pink" (Lychnis

---

[11] One can compare the earth organism with the three–membered human organism and assign the tropics to the metabolic region, the poles to the sensory, nervous system in the head and the temperate zones in between to the rhythmic system.

viscaria) exudes its sticky, blackish violet resin. This will be effective against excessive sulfuric (inflammatory metabolic) processes in the human rhythmic system, i.e., in the "carbon organ", the lungs.

Another process that is involved here becomes manifest in a higher silica content in some species and in a higher iron content in others. Thereby one has more of a relation to the skin and sense organs in the plants with silica, and to the blood and breathing process in the ones with iron, which becomes manifest in the saponin process in pinks.

Vitaceae – Grape family

The plants in the grape family are a present of the cosmos to the earth which the cosmos has given in a special way and the earth has received in a particular way. The human beings who were created by the earth have also received these plants as something that helped them to go through a particular phase in their development, but that also became a danger. Bread and wine, wheat and grapevine stand before us as symbols of human nutrition and as the members of the plant kingdom that give us food; the first has an Apollonian nature and the second a Dionysian one. The two substances starch and sugar arise from the primal part of plant formation, the assimilation process that unites the stream of cosmic light and warmth in the green leaf with the water that streams up from the earth and with the surrounding ocean of air. Grain seeds make more starch, and fruits and berries make more sugar.

One could hardly think of a greater contrast than that between a grain field and a vineyard. Here one has strictly upright stems with narrow, linear leaves and ears that are borne upwards and there arbitrarily wandering, playfully winding and grasping, leaf hands that spread out horizontally with rampantly swelling and heavily hanging grapes. In grains the earthly element is carried up into the light, and in grapevines something cosmic goes down and loses itself in the earthly element. The construction of grains shows a sacred soberness and that of a grapevine a playful fantasy. Goethe referred to the vertical and spiral tendencies in plants, and it is clear that the first is present in grains and the second in grapevines.

Let's take a look at the whole family first in order to get an overview of the formative motif in this particular plant type. It is divided into over 600 species, most of them vines in warm and tropical regions that wind around their supports and hang on with tendrils or with grippers. In the large tropical genus Cissus one gets thick, fleshy, cactus-like stems that remind one of the Queen of the Night or similar jointed cactuses, or of swollen leaves, trunks, roots and burls; or the leaves atrophy and change and appear as thick, green winged stems whose shoots have been held back. This tendency towards watery swellings that shows up as the formation of large, juicy berries tells one a great deal. One would say that the flowering process is quite active here but individual flowers are small and not showy, with greenish whitish yellows, and their wonderful, sweet and dry fragrances attracts more attention than their colors do. The flower petals often stand out like caps since their tips are grown together.

What mainly interests us here is the Vitis genus with over 40 species that have spread out over the warmer parts of the northern temperate zone, from North America over Europe and Asia in China, Korea and Japan, and new species are being developed everywhere.

Vitis vinifera, the European wine grape, is cultivated in all of the earth's warm, temperate regions. This is a plant whose cultivation, harvesting and pressing is depicted on ancient Egyptian monuments, and one can still encounter its wild form in woods along the large rivers of Southern Europe and in Asia Minor, in the Mediterranean region, around the Black Sea, in the Caucasus mountains, Crimea, Northern Persia and along the Rhine and the Danube. This Vitis vinifera, variation sylvestris, sends its roots deep down into the ground and climbs up trees. Some were found that went up approximately 100 feet, and its vines can be 20 inches in diameter. The berries remain bean-sized but can get quite sweet if it is hot enough. The plants in our vineyards on five or six foot supports don't show much of this tremendous growing power but one can see more of it in the vines that grow up elms and mulberry trees in northern Italy, and in the ones that cover our house walls. However a lot of this vegetative power has gone into the exuberant berry formation. Growers have selectively bred and cultivated almost countless variations of this meadow vine that has become an expression of the climates and landscapes in which they've grown. Every difference in the hill's angle to the sun, and in the proximity of waters that reflect and store the sun's warmth, changes the sweetness and flavoring of the berries and gives the pressed berry juice a different taste. It is almost too cold for grapevines north of the Alps today, and it is only the tireless efforts and care of growers that keep them in the vineyards that have obviously gotten colder since the Middle Ages. Just look at all the vineyards at the upper ends of South

German river valleys which have been abandoned. And gardeners have to protect the grapes that are still growing from a host of molds and insects that always attack things that aren't very vital anymore. Rudolf Steiner once said that green houses were the only place north of the Alps where one could grow healthy grapevines.

However, even a healthy vine is connected with lower fungus life that is waiting to develop and destroy what the vine has produced. We are referring to the yeast spores that are on grapeskins. Every kind of grape vine has its own kind of ferment which sits passively on the skins, but storms into action as soon as the grapes are squashed and their juice is pressed out. One can transfer these yeasts to sugar solutions, and the resulting artificial wines will be remotely similar to the ones that one gets by fermenting grapes.

Thus something hovers around grapes that wants to ferment them. This outer readiness to ferment is also met by an inner process to a greater extent than in any other plant. Rudolf Steiner gave the key to an understanding of the nature of the grape vine, which in fact expresses its secret and makes its role in human evolution comprehensible. He said the following about it in lecture one of the *Effect of Occult Development upon Man's Sheathes and His Self*: "If we look at plants we see that they all reach a certain point in their organization, with the exception of the grape vine, which goes beyond this. What other plants save up for their young, all the germinating power that is otherwise saved up for the young germ and doesn't pour into the rest of the plant, all this pours into the flesh of grapes in a certain way."

Thus we are told that the relation between the seed and the fruit of a grape vine is different than in other plants. One can see the spatial manifestations of a plant's live formative forces body, expansion and contraction, at every stage of its growth. The sprout shoots out of the constricted seed, gathers itself together in the node, expands in the leaf, contracts in the calyx, opens up in the flower, condenses into a seed and swells up in the fruit. The growth and unfolding forces in a seed are pulled together into a point that has become hidden from the senses. They have withdrawn into a real, super spatial, super temporal realm and have only left a copy of themselves behind, into which they will enter again when the seed germinates. This super-spatial realm is the ocean of formative forces and life that envelops the earth in an etheric sheath and is identical with the etheric world, whereas the fruit is a last material, spatial expansion of the plant. The substances that have been deposited in it have been permanently separated from the plant's life. On the other hand, the substances in a seed are taken hold of by the germ, broken down and then taken up into the life of the seedling. Now yeast fungi treat the substances in the grape in the same way that the seedling treats the seed's substances; they break it down and thereby develop the tremendous sprouting power that ferments the berry juice in a stormy way. Everything has been prepared in the berry so that this tremendous sprouting power can be unleashed. However, this discharge permits a lower, formless, fungous life to develop but not that of the grapevine.

Thereby alcohol arises out of the sugar that has been formed by cosmic sun forces. However, this poisonous substance paralyzes the life that formed it and eventually kills it. Thus the ferment develops a very paradoxical biological process, one that terminates and eliminates itself. Thereby the fermentation product is conserved and mummified and it becomes a wine that keeps.

Grape juice and all things that contain sugar are important food stuffs for human beings, so important that humans prepare this sugar themselves by digesting starchy foods such as bread fruits. They convert this sugar into the body sugar that circulates in the blood and enters into the tissues in muscles and nerves, and in short is and must be present everywhere in the human organism. The latter maintains the temperature and the sugar content of its blood with equal care. Man's highest member, his I and spiritual core, needs this sugar in order to develop its impulses in the body. "Grape sugar is a substance that can work in the sphere of the I organization." "The I organization is present wherever sugar is present; when sugar arises the I organization appears and humanizes the subhuman (vegetative, animal) body." "As the blood and its sugar content circulates through the whole body, it also carries the I organization through it." (Rudolf Steiner/Ita Wegman, M.D., *Fundamentals of Therapy*, Chap. 8).

Sugar formation in plants is brought about by cosmic forces that represent the plants' I region. They work from the sun towards the earth's center, as we have already pointed out a number of times in this *Healing Plants*. Of course, whatever is created by cosmic I forces has a special relationship with the human I.

Why doesn't the sugar in a person's body ferment if it does so everywhere outside of it? Why doesn't alcohol arise in the human body?

These are questions that one has to ask oneself. Rudolf Steiner answered them on the basis of his spiritual scientific investigations. The activities and organizing power of a person's higher members, mainly the I, keep the fermentation process away from one's organization, especially from the upper one. It is true that traces of alcohol are formed in the lower organization to hold the physical organization together and to serve a certain mineralization and preservation of the organ's protein processes. The latter have to be protected against what immediately happens to protein when it is separated from the body (it decomposes and its form disintegrates).

Anyone who takes in alcohol from outside disrupts these delicate processes. Alcohol takes the power to control carbohydrate processes away from the I, or what one rightly calls one's self; the power to control carbohydrate processes puts itself in its place as a kind of "counter-I." Ethanol fermentation forces usurp the I's control at the place where it develops consciousness and directs the will. For alcohol, this sugar derivative circumvents the digestive paths prescribed for other substances, and enters the blood directly. It presses into the sense organs, organs of consciousness, and the whole upper organization, and befuddles them and thereby cuts its host off from the outer world, since it drives the I out of the upper person. It diverts the I towards the lower organization, which is made more physical, coarser and more cohesive. The spiritual core thereby becomes much more tightly connected with the physical body than nature intended. A person intoxicated by alcohol behaves the way he does on account of his own body, which is experienced in a more powerful way than a sober person does. Alcohol constrains the spiritual member, the I, to go down into the body completely and thus preventing connection to their spiritual origins in this way. Alcohol intoxication thus increases the egotistical forces. A drunk enjoys himself, relates everything to himself and in an intoxicated state, eventually sinks completely into the body.

Quite a few millennia ago this cutting off from the spiritual world, development of egotistical focus and experiencing of one's self on one's own physical body was a world process that was necessary for mankind's development towards independence. It was promoted by the consumption of alcoholic beverages. The grapevine had a mission in human evolution and civilization, and wine was offered as a cultic drink in certain mystery centers where Dionysius was worshipped as a divine teacher of man. He killed off the old clairvoyant powers and he intoxicated man so that he would dare to go into the sensory, physical, material world, where he encountered himself and his fellows as the crown of creation and the god of the earth. One still finds a particularly heavy use of alcohol today in tribes which had retained "second sight" and other atavistic clairvoyant powers until fairly recently, and who wanted to get rid of them.

The forces of the lower, body-bound I, or egoism, have been developed enough today; people have become completely cut off from the reality of the spiritual world and have lost the knowledge of the higher I that experiences itself as a spiritual being in a spiritual world. A further advance on this path would not be progress, it would be harmful. A person who is seeking one's true being today must open up the portals to the spiritual world again, and must have the will to develop the senses for its perception. A person must understand that one is a spiritual being here during life on earth, and not just after death. The grapevine's mission is over, to the extent that it is a giver of wine.

And oddly enough, the grapevine's vitality has been declining for about 80 years already. A host of pests has attacked it, there is practically no end to sprayings in the vineyard, and the outfits that gardeners wear in their vineries are increasingly reminiscent of soldiers' protective gear in poison gas warfare. Even so, grapevines are becoming ever more sick and susceptible to disease. One can foresee a time when this cultivated plant will no longer be of any importance as such.

A technological age requires much more alert and well-functioning senses, a sense of reality, and a soul attitude that develops and cultivates objectivity. All of these things are incompatible with the consumption of alcohol. People who want to dissipate the fog of materialistic delusions, enter the clear light of spiritual reality, and take hold of the higher I, will avoid alcohol, for it disrupts one's power to perceive spiritual things. Social goals that are appropriate for our time can only be attained if people get out of the confining confusion of their lower, selfish Is and find a way into the real nature of other human beings, so that their self-love is overcome and a real love for one's neighbors arises. The people who set themselves such goals will have to give up their love of alcohol.

This is required by the threefold nature of our time.

*

The Dionysius cult has come to an end. It has been replaced by the being who said: I am the grapevine and you are the shoots. He is the leader who enables us to overcome the lower I and to find the higher one. The higher I no longer needs a development of egoistical forces, it experiences a strengthening of its nature through its connection with the Christ Being, in Whom the self receives the power to become selfless without losing itself. An age whose people place the forces of nature at His service, search for the spirit and want to build new social forms will have to become a Christian age because of its threefold nature.

*

Water, warmth and carbohydrate processes live in the grapevine in a special way. Their characteristics are quite similar to those of the human liver process. This gives one an idea about the healing possibilities of Vitis vinifera. Rudolf Steiner recommended a new remedy for malfunctioning livers that is prepared from the leaves of strawberries and grapes. (See Volume I of this Healing Plants for a discussion of strawberries and their pharmaceutical possibilities.) Carbohydrates are produced in grape leaves, and transformed sugars fill the berries. The leaves contain 2% sugar, which is quite a lot for a leaf, and inositol (a fully hydroxylated derivative of cyclohexane with the same empirical formula as grape sugar $C_6H_{12}C_6$). Inositol combines easily with phosphoric acid (making phytic acid) and it plays an important part in the metabolism of the liver and of muscles. Therefore it is an important substance not only for plant life (for instance, it is found in seeds together with phosphorus) but also for people. Inositol stimulates the liver's action energetically and it gets phosphorus involved in the fat process.

The plant acids in grape leaves indicate the presence of certain congestions in the plant's life which it has to overcome through its interaction with the earth's substances. The reader will find a more detailed discussion of this in connection with what was said about plant acids in the sections on cactuses, stonecrops, sorrels and rues. Therefore sluggish abdominal action, hindrances to healthy metabolic activity and a tendency towards hardening and mineralization in the liver and gall bladder region are also combated by the above mentioned preparation from grape leaves.

Grape leaves also contain waxes, choline (which also stimulates liver action strongly), 5–7% mineral salts (including quite a lot of sodium salts), and more boron than one ordinarily finds in plants. Boron's properties are between those of silica and sulfur, and it is present in all plants that produce a lot of sugar; there is quite a lot of it in flower nectars, and so it obviously has something to do with the process that drives the sugar in leaves into the flowers in a centrifugal manner.

Honeysuckles – Caprifoliaceae

The honeysuckle or goat's leaf family that is botanically similar to the larger madder family (Rubiaceae) mainly chooses the temperate zone for its more than 350 species. It forms shrubs and small trees with wood that is sometimes bonehard but also often with soft, airy and dry pith in the branches and young twigs. It fills these plants with tenacious, powerfully shooting life, and they rapidly cover even poor and rocky soils. They have plenty of leaves, most of which are opposite, undivided. Some are lobed. A few are like maple leaves, and only those of the elderberries are compound pinnate. One often finds glands which secrete nectar on the leaves, which probably arose from transformed accessory leaves; thus the sugar process even drips sweets out of the leaf region. This attracts a lot of ants and plant lice, and one often finds galls on the leaves. Caterpillars and gall flies even live in flowers (which then fail to open).

The flowering process develops sumptuously with bright reddish, yellowish and white shades of color, sweet, and even intoxicating scents. There is no shortage of ornamental plants here (honeysuckle, snowberry, weigela, viburnum), but a certain toxic element runs through the whole family. The juicy reddish yellow, red, black and blue berries or cherrylike pitted fruits that emerge from inferior ovaries can induce diarrhea and vomiting. Thus we become aware of a powerful astral impact. The flowers form in a twofold way, sturdy, erect, treelike plants produce wide umbrellas, with many small, symmetrical, wide open, flat flowers (e.g. elderberry, viburnum), whereas the swaying plants that tend to wind around things have beautiful, large, one–sidedly symmetrical flowers sometimes with a separate underlip (honeysuckle).

Three of the 21 species of elder grow in European regions: Sambucus nigra, Sambucus racemosa,and Sambucus ebulus (black fruited, red fruited and dwarf elders). Viburnum or snowball has 125 species in Europe, Asia and North America. They are woody plants with flexible stalks; some of them wind around things. They decorate themselves with large umbrellas, consisting of many flowers at the end of the stems. Viburnum lantana, the wayfaring tree, with black, stone berries grows on rocky limestone soils; Highbush Cranberry Viburnum opulus, with a wreath of large, border flowers around the white umbrellas, and red fruits, grows in damp woods and bushy areas. The berries and bark of v. opulus v. prunifolia, which smell like valerian and are purgative and emetic, have been used for threatened abortions and dysmenorrhea. Of about ten Linnaeus species, the dainty twin flower, linnaea borealis, dares to go far north; pairs of little white bells that smell like vanilla rise up out of the leaf axils of trailing stems with small leaves; the insides of the bells are streaked with red. The plant is small, its hardiness and its many flowers show that it is a caprifolium through and through. One should also mention Symphoricarpos racemosus, or snowberry, which originally came from the Pacific Northwest although it has been growing in Europe for some time now. (Children love to crunch the glossy, airy, white berries in the fall.) It has long stalks and short racemes of pink flowers at their ends; its root and berries have a diuretic, purging effect and one uses extracts from them to combat nausea and vomiting during pregnancy.

Lonicera, honeysuckle, or the real goats leaf (caprifoliaceae) has about 120 species including many climbing ones with flower clusters; the erect ones decorate themselves with pairs of flowers on a common stem. The tubular flowers as in Lonicera fragrant issima and other species give out seductive smells.

By and large the caprifoliaceae are vigorous but strongly astralized plants. Because of their intensive flowering activity their action is directed towards the metabolic region and the astral body's activities there. A look at the family's most important medicinal plant elderberry will reveal more details about this.

Sambucus nigra – Elderberry, Pipe Tree

One can see indestructible life in the powerful way the European elder takes hold on the rockiest soil, in dumps, cracks in walls, and rocks in ruins, and in the way it springs up again no matter how often its stems are cut down to the roots or are otherwise injured. It puts out long, very green and juicy shoots each year, which lignify slowly, although they only condense to airy, white pith inside, which is a characteristic feature of the honeysuckle family. The broad, pinnately compound leaves are soft and plastic; the shrub looks like it is hydrophilic, and in fact, it looks for semi-shaded places at the edge of the woods so that it can flourish, suck in the soil's moisture energetically and exhale it out into the air again. That is why its torn off leaves wilt rapidly. The sap is very sugary and it often attracts legions of black plant lice that suck at the plentiful sweets and thereby attract ants, who also find nectar on the plant elsewhere, and namely in 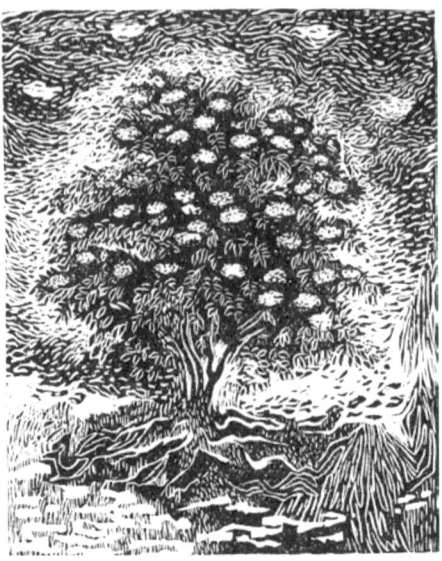 nectarines that were formed out of threadlike accessory leaves that are not in the flower regions but are one level lower.

Once one has become aware of the pipe tree's sprouting power one could ask: why doesn't it grow into a tall tree rather than just a small one or a big bush? This is obviously due to the forces that split the shoot into branches after its initial rapid growth, which then run into broad umbels where the growth atomizes into countless small, white flowery stars. Just as the circumference crosses a circle's radius perpendicularly, so the surface of the umbrella of flowers, an image of the spherical heavens, limits the radial sprouting power of the shoot.

However, the leaves are already preparing for what is disclosed in these many clusters of flowers. They take abnormally strong warmth effects into their shaded, moist, juicy herbaceous sphere. If one crushes a leaf, one smells something like smoldering wet wood or fire that has had water thrown on it. One could also be reminded of the smell of sweat. What is working in here in an abnormal way produces poisons, just as in a number of other caprifolios, namely glycosides that split off hydrocyanic acid. Thus we run into the same cyanide process that develops in the ripening of bitter almonds through an "inner combustion". (See Volume 1) One can produce this process artificially by heating proteins in the absence of air. What occurs in the seed process of bitter almond trees has a preliminary stage in elderberries in their leaves.

In the summer, after our plant has heated itself up in its leaves for awhile, the overly strong flowering process steams out of the warmed, moist element of the fully grown leaves. It is really sweated out. When the flowers first open they smell etheric and fresh, but they soon acquire their characteristic sweaty, sulfurous and aromatic odor. Some think that an especially large number of flowers is a sign that the following winter will be harsh. If the blossom's water is removed through drying or baking in dough they give out a familiar, pleasing, salutary fragrance. The flowers produce a large amount of sulfurous yellow pollen.

The flowers then develop into juicy, purplish blackberries. Thus the fluidic organization participates in their formation and there is no drying out in the fruit region. As sweet as these berries are, there is something watery, cold and unpleasant about their taste, and one gets an inkling of something in Caprifoliceas that induces diarrhea and vomiting. They must be well cooked with sugar and spiced with cinnamon and cloves to please one's palate and stomach.

A dark element permeates the whole plant, as one can see from the withering, blackish leaves and the black fruits. Isn't the elderberry like an image of healing nature force that brings out a dark, cold element out of the soil's moisture, masters it, warms it up and sweats it out in the following process?

In a lecture Rudolf Steiner gave to doctors on April 17, 1921 (*Anthroposophical Spiritual Science and Medical Therapy*, Mercury Press), he described the elderberry as follows: "Let's look at . . .where the flower effect . . . becomes particularly manifest . . .where many small flowers become an inflorescence, as in elderberry or pipe tree, Sambucus nigra. We should realize that precisely those forces shoot into the plant here that have a lot to do with the earth's environment and that contain cosmic influences and currents. We note this from the fact that elderberry flowers also contain essential oils. But we particularly note this from the fact that elderberry flowers contain sulfur. "This sulfur that is carried by flower processes strongly stimulates the human etheric body that is active in the fluidic organization. The etheric body strives towards aeration and to being taken hold of by aeration, by breathing processes and therewith by the astral body's activity. The astral body's activity is stimulated indirectly through the etheric activity and so is the breathing in the upper, rear organs, but not so much in the head organs as in those that belong to actual respiration." (ibid)

The stimulation of breathing also stimulates the blood circulation, which can counteract a number of metabolic effects, promote the elimination and perspiration and work against coughing and rheumatic processes. (See the discussion about sulfur processes in Cruciferae and lilies in Volume 1.)

Whereas the sphere of activity described above essentially agrees with previous medical experiences if not with previous explanations, the medical use of elderberry pith is something new. Rudolf Steiner recommended its use, together with a flower infusion, in a case where the activities of the etheric and astral bodies were insufficiently harmonized, which became manifest in disrupted waking up and falling asleep processes and abnormal perspiration. The gentle diuretic effect of elderberry flowers combined with the porosity of its pith could be of help here.

Thus the very element intervenes particularly deeply in the development of elder pith, that is, into the realm of wood formation, solids and the life ether, and not just into the leaves and fluid processes or the region of the chemical ether. Now that many examples of the way air moves through the plant in connection with astralization processes have been given, the reader will be able to figure out what happens in this case alone. It is rather strange that the elderberry produces a kind of solid foam at the place where other plants grow wood.

Sea Buckthorn – Hippophaë Rhamnoides

Images of a Plant's Essential Nature and Therapeutic Imaginations

One can be sure that doctors will become interested in a plant if the analytical work of a chemist shows that it contains this or that active ingredient. Such plants suddenly begin to make an impression on people and from this viewpoint Sea Buckthorn is a very impressive plant, since its Vitamin C content exceeds that of any other plant that has been analyzed so far.

And yet our knowledge of the connections between medicinal plants and human beings is moved into the chemical laboratory and away from a vivid perception of them through an approach that is only interested in active ingredients. No doubt valuable things are found in this way. However, over and beyond such analytical results a doctor will want to have a direct way of looking at things that will open up insights into the natural processes that can stimulate healing processes in humans. Therefore, we will try to give an idea of how sea buckthorn expresses its own nature, which includes a lot more than just being the number one source of Vitamin C. This comprehensive nature must also be able to tell us why this plant produces so much Vitamin C and also carotene or provitamin A.

If each doctor gets images of the true nature of plants encountered, one's therapeutic imagination will be able to enkindled directly. They have quite a different power than do abstract thoughts about Nature. The therapist's will to heal that was enkindled by his picture of the patient can, as it were, take hold of such pictures that should be elaborated by the knowers of plants, and can take the things out of nature that can become remedies. Thus such images of each plant's essential nature will be very important to doctors, and they will see that form of botany in them that is in accordance with their profession.

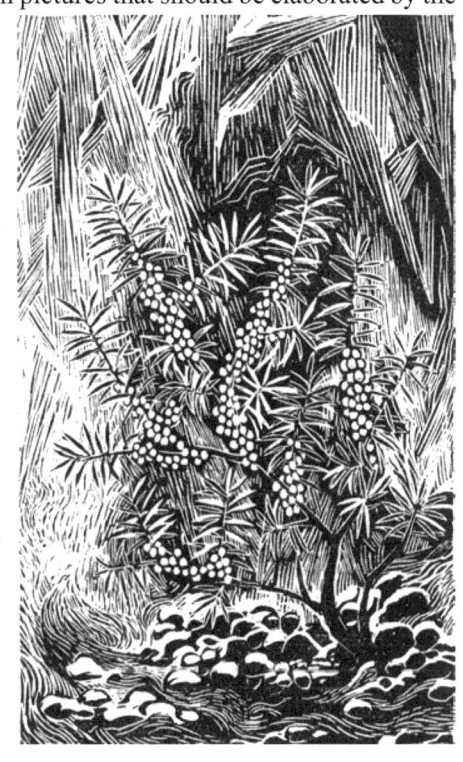

(One already learns quite a lot about sea buckthorn from the fact that it grows on the sterile sand dunes of European sea coasts and high up into the north, on the gravely banks of alpine's brooks and rivers and on the rockiest waste lands, as the first pioneer of life. It creates the humus which other, more demanding plants need, and it immediately disappears when the land that has been brought back to life by it, begins to get too shady from all the new plants and bushes. For although sea buckthorn is insensitive to extreme poor soil around its root region, it is very demanding with respect to light; the latter must be available to it at its full intensity. It likes small bare gravel or sand that is loose, airy and moistened by moving water (no congested water will do) in short, a mobile, airy soil with fresh water seeping through. Its connections with water are expressed in its names, sea thorn, Rhine thorn, and its connection with soil in the names sand thorn and gravel thorn.

Sea buckthorn sends runners from the roots in all directions and puts up new shoots from them, and thereby giving expression to an untameable vitality in its subterranean organs. However, as soon as it shoots up into the realm of air, light, warmth and cosmic radiations, a great change occurs in the plant's life that flows towards all sides in the mineral, solid and fluidic regions. Here its life forces become introverted rather than extroverted. This becomes manifest in the many thorns that stick out of all shoots, branches, twigs and side shoots. Sea buckthorn puts out long, short and very short skewers in all directions. The impulse of the formative forces body, that super physical member that permeates physical substantiality with life, is withdrawn and dammed up in its thorn formation. They pull back and don't become manifest in the original direction anymore. They become available to the terminal side buds that shoot out strongly and take over the main shoot's task. It is as if the main stem of a spruce or other tree gets lopped off, in which case its strength shoots into the side branches.

This is how the strange, seemingly erratic branching of sea buckthorn comes about; each main shoot forks into four or five side shoots below the end thorn, which go through something similar after they have grown for awhile. The new shoots put out small, narrow leaves that are shiny and silvery underneath. Second year shoots don't put out side twigs anymore, but only short shoots, and they get thicker until they become branches. Sea buckthorn rays its life out into the periphery in this way and rigidifies inside it in thorns and lances; when it gets old its growth pattern can look like that of an umbrella pine. However, this umbrella out at the periphery is a very illuminated zone, and our plant drives its whole life into it and leaves withered wood inside it. The green and silvery canopy of leaves spreads out in this zone in an airy way, which never gets so thick that light and air would be unable to illumine and play around the whole shrub right down to the ground. As the sea buckthorn continues to grow it pulls its life into ever wider spheres of light. It wants a great deal of light so it can literally bathe in it, and it receives it from two sides in the places where it grows, directly and indirectly by reflection from the water surfaces it likes to grow near. However, sea buckthorn quickly disappears if willows and other plants grow up and cast their shadows over it, because it doesn't really like that. But it really likes wind, and so its super structure is built into air and light to quite a large extent.

This also comes to expression in its flowering process. This is divided into "male" and "female" bushes and it surrenders itself to the wind that mediates between the two. The flower buds that develop on the annual growths are carried through the winter and unfold in April, especially when the weather is windy and dry. The flowers are plain and primitively formed, adapted entirely to wind pollination, formed by the wind and for the wind, and are closely connected with the element of light and air. The female flower doesn't lose its sheath, it grows around the little carpel, becomes fleshy and thereby forms yellowish red pseudo fruit, the sea buckthorn berry which therefore is a pseudo berry. Here we're really eating transformed flowers. The fruits are usually taken by crows, magpies and grackles, and the seeds germinate quickly in warm, late spring days and grow into 20 inch shoots with about 4 inch side shoots in the first year. Growth is slower thereafter and at best the plant becomes a small thorn tree, with very hard wood. Sea buckthorns begin to bear fruit after about five years. But what doesn't get very tall gets that much wider as stems shoot up from horizontal roots, and after awhile one can have a small grove from one plant, that is divided into old, withering little trees at the center, vigorous shrubs around them laden with berries and new shoots coming out of the ground in the outer circle.

Thus sea buckthorn obviously has strong connections with light above ground. However, the connections are already stimulated in its roots, and namely by the silica rich ground. Silica's reaction to light has often been described in this Healing Plants from a number of different sides. One finds a number of finely opened up, attenuated siliceous materials in the treasure trove of medications in anthroposophic extended medicine. They especially have an enlivening and shaping effect on the sensory sphere that is represented by the eye or light organ. Very finely dispersed silica is always available to the roots of sea buckthorn, for it is constantly being put into the water by a kind of natural potentization process where rock fragments grind each other to powder as they are moved by running water. Such silicic acid becomes vividly manifest in sea buckthorn's shape, for the latter enables one to see some of the relations between the silica (which is really mineralized luminosity) and light. The plant form's life dynamics are both crystalline rigidity and life that is active entirely in light; it flees that dark, counterplayer of silica in the soil, humus, which gives plants more substantially massive bodies. It would rather stand entirely on the side of formative forces and have nothing to do with substance forces.

Once one begins to understand the fine interaction between minerals, water, air and light that builds up and shapes sea buckthorn, it becomes clear that this interaction can occur best in the mountains, and that the best qualities of sea buckthorn berries can be brought out by the Alpine valleys in southern Switzerland, for example. (And in fact, analysis shows that berries from there have the most vitamins.)

This is the place to go into the substances that are found in its fruits. They are interesting in themselves, but even more so because they point to the formative processes that produced them. For it is possible to get a rational insight into the way a healing substance can intervene in the living contest of forces in the human being, and can initiate healing processes, from the connection between the formative process and the substance that is formed by it.

One should first mention carotene, which gives the berries their bright orange red color. Carotene is present in many plants and is visible in the yellow and yellowish red colors of their flowers, in the pigments in red and yellow fruits like the tomato. It is hidden by the chlorophyll in leaves and it is in some roots like that of the carrot, which gave this substance its name. The hidden carotene in the leaves becomes clearly manifest in the fall, when chlorophyll disappears.

Carotene is a real "light substance"; its task in plants is to absorb light energies and to transfer them to chlorophyll. It becomes visible in the ripening fruits as they shed their green. The large quantity in which it is formed is an expression of the strong intervention of light in the formation of plants. Carotene is the provitamin A that is converted into vitamin A in the human organism. A deficient amount of it shows up as a devitalization and desiccation of the ectoderm and of all the organs that proceed from it and turn towards the outside. This is a primary sphere of action for silicic acid. Vitamin A concentrates at the rear of the eyes and in visual purple; a lack of it leads to night blindness.

The carotene content of sea buckthorn berries is an expression of the great part that silicic acid processes and light dynamics play in the life of the plant that bears them.

Sea Buckthorn berry juice also contains up to 2% fatty oils, and the seed has about 12%. Oil palms and the olive tree are some of the few other plants that permeate their fruit is flesh with fatty oil, and not just the seeds. That is quite an unusual achievement at our latitudes. It tells us something about the particularly strong sucking in of cosmic forces of light and warmth that distinguishes our plant. The biologically so valuable unsaturated fatty acids that have a vitamin character, linoleic, linolenic, and isolinoleic acids are present in this oil. This points to the special kind of etheric formative forces that are peculiar to our plants. One finds a lot of such unsaturated fatty acid in poppies, flax, rape and other plants that grow in northern regions; their formation is connected with a predominance of cosmic forces over earth forces. (The saturated, inactive, hydrogenated acids predominate in tropical fats.) Thus the special nature of sea buckthorn also becomes manifest in its fat metabolism.

Sea buckthorn berries also contain a lot of malic acid, and other acids arise when sugars are oxidized and exhaled. If oxygen can unfold its activity without hindrances, sugar is broken down into carbon dioxide and water. (Its activity always has to do with the intervention of live etheric formative forces into the physical; the more intensive the life is the more energetic the aeration is.) If life is congested, the aeration also gets held up and only goes halfway to completion. This shows up especially in the succulent leaves of stone crop plants, the bodies of cactuses, etc. Juicy fruits are also watery and succulent. In fruit acids one can almost taste the battle of life against congestive influences, and in sea buckthorn the latter comes from its sterile growing places.

Another plant acid is Vitamin C or L–ascorbic acid, which is closely related to citric acid. We find a lot of it in plants that have to deal intensively with congestions of life forces; for instance, in scurvy grass. Rudolf Steiner described the essential nature of this plant that likes to grow along salty northern sea coasts as follows. Through its sulfur process it heals and accelerates its own sluggish protein metabolism that is conditioned by its unfavorable growing places (dead, sandy soil, salt content and cold).[12] Sea buckthorn has to deal with similarly unfavorable conditions, and it is helped by aeration, much light and the silicic acid in the ground, whose dynamics it takes into its formation. (It is interesting that

---

[12] Rudolf Steiner, *Spiritual Science and Medicine*, Lecture 15

dog rose is another vigorous thorn bush that also likes much light, takes up intensive silicic acid processes with the formation of its seeds, loves high mountains, and contains the second highest amount of Vitamin C in the plants that have been analyzed so far. However, rose hips themselves only have half the amount of Vitamin C that is in sea buckthorn fruits. The dog rose takes strong light and formative forces into its life processes also.)

Every plant feeds itself in two ways, out of the dark earth realm, and out of the atmosphere that is irradiated and illuminated by cosmic forces. However, some plant species emphasize one or the other of these ways. There are plants that demand or draw on much humus, and others that demand a great deal from the cosmos and very little from the ground. Sea buckthorn definitely belongs to the latter group, for it requires practically nothing from the ground and a maximum from the light realm.

Humans also need things from the earth and forces from the cosmos to build up their bodies. Until now, focus has been mainly on investigation of the first kind of nutrition. However, investigators are gradually becoming aware that nutrition has a cosmic, formative forces side that is just as important as the material one. For some time now, there have been many indications to this effect in the medicine that has been extended by the cognitional methods of spiritual science.[13] A lack of light is just as detrimental to the human organism as too little fat. If this cosmic nourishment decreases, as in the short days of winter or because of pathological situations, etc., and the symptoms that are generally considered to be due to a lack of Vitamin C arise, sea buckthorn preparations are available so that doctors can combat the extensive causes. Sea Buckthorn and the preparations that are gained from it will also be welcome as preventives, accessories to therapeutic measures, and convalescing agents when the "cosmic qualities" in foods decrease due to seasonal fluctuations or when foods are grown for their bulk rather than for quality.

E. O. Eckstein wrote something similar about sea buckthorn berries in 1943, and then he said, "On the basis of these observations and deliberations we have added Hippophae rhamnoides to the many plants that we process. We have seen that it keeps the promise of what the whole

---

[13] Friedr. Husemann, Stuttgart 1951

picture of its real nature indicates. If carefully prepared the juice keeps its strong effect much longer than any similar natural product. And the effect of its forces is that an organism whose tone has been reduced will be reinvigorated. It can alleviate and often eliminate tiredness, fatigue states and everything that one can call deficiency ailments today (where in many cases no outer deficiency is present)."

Vitamins

The living essence of a plant has to be comprehended step by step. At the first level we grasp it through our senses and we experience its scent, colors, taste, softness and solidity. At the second level we elaborate the sense impressions with our thinking and we become aware of the plant's shape and substances. We cannot remain here, we get a step further by becoming aware of the change in form and transformation of substances that become manifest in growth, disintegration, coming to life and dying. Here a surprise element or something essential shines through the phenomenal forms; its perception requires one to reach the highest level, and for this one needs the power to see the being. The higher senses that are required for this develop as one climbs up from one stage to the next. Inner spiritual organs of perception develop through exercise, if one follows the phenomena of developing and withering life and the real essence that reveals and conceals itself with strong soul forces, inner participation and constant effort.[14]

If one wants to understand plant life and its processes one has to take inner and outer perception together, and physical and spiritual perception must work together. This is particularly true if one follows the material nature or the material side of plants. One has to be very careful here. For the methods which chemists arrive at by working with dead substances must destroy, divide and kill plants so that they fall apart into thousands of different kinds of substances that can be identified in a chemical way. The only thing that can be chemically established and grasped in a living plant is what it separates from its life stream. But what is pulled or thrown out of the ocean of life onto the beach of death is obviously no longer life. It is just as much of a corpse as the fish which the low tide left behind on

---

[14] See Rudolf Steiner, *How Does One Attain Knowledge of Higher Worlds?*

the beach. One should never forget this, otherwise we will have a very deceptive picture of the plant world. A plant does not consist of the substances that have been pulled out of the stream of life. It is true that this stream takes in substances and throws out, but what gets into the flow of life in between absorption and expulsion has stripped off the material properties that it has from its earth connections. It has been taken in by higher force realms and completely transformed, as we pointed out in the introduction to Volume I of this *Healing Plants*.

Thus forewarned, one can speak about protein s, carbohydrates, fats, essential oils, glycosides, alkaloids, etc., and about plant substances or substances which plants make available to us in quantities that can be weighed and touched as foods, gourmet foods and remedies. The latter's quality is all the better the more recently they have been taken out of the life stream. All of these substances become denatured, and then they spoil, some faster and others slower, depending on whether they were formed in the middle of the life stream or more at its edge. As the substances become denatured they approach the condition that our modern chemists can grasp, put into formulas and synthesize.

However, humans and animals can get very sick, if one tries to feed them artificial mixtures of polypeptides, triglycerides of fatty acids and carbohydrates, just because one thinks that food consists of them. Such voluntary or involuntary experiments made people realize that humans have always eaten whole fruits, vegetables, milk, cheese, honey, bread, fish and other meat and not on proteins, fats and carbohydrates. This showed them very forcefully that there is a hidden activity in living substances that cannot be grasped in a coarse material way. However, since scientists didn't want to change their customary way of investigating things, they just discovered a new class of finer substances, consisting of vitamins, hormones and biocatalysts, which can be obtained from plants in a much more finely divided state than proteins, fats and carbohydrates and with which one can regulate growth and life processes in an amazing way with only minimal doses. So does the secret of life have a material nature after all? Or did one arrive at a material lever from which life is created and directed? Initially, one spoke of vitamins, etc., for example, vitamins A, B, C, D, E, F, H, K and so on.

Now that chemists have come up with their formulas one speaks of ascorbic acid, thiamine, etc. It is odd that these substances are used in organisms in such a highly diluted form and that they have this in common with the traces of boron, manganese, molybdenum, zinc, vanadium and others that the organism needs just as much. In all of these, large effects are connected with almost vanishing amounts of substances as in homeopathy. Whereas one weighs kilograms of proteins, fats and carbohydrates, the standard of measurement in the realm of trace elements is the microgram, or the millionth part of a gram.

Thus some of the substances that form out of an organism's weaving forces are material, coarse and ponderable while others that are also connected with important life functions only condense out of this weaving of forces in a delicate way and just barely become manifest in the material world. Coarse materials and fine materials come to meet us. A plant presents the coarse materials in its physical body to our senses, whereas its fine substances are connected with biological control functions and with the body of formative forces or etheric body. The latter controls certain processes in the gross materials through the instrument of the fine materials.

Let's take a brief look at the coarse substantiality of a plant. Living protein is basically the primal and basic substance, the living water and plastic, primal substance in whose womb all other substances arise, both coarse and fine ones. The leaves' chloroplasts and dyes arise from it, they are formed by light and for light dynamics and become active in a two dimensional plane. The dyes include the chlorophyll which produces the carbohydrates starch and sugar, and carotene, which is converted to vitamin A in the human organism and which has to do with the absorption of light in plants.

The carbohydrates that form in this leafy region do not become ponderable, for they are immediately transformed in the life stream in various ways. The coarse and material things that appear are ones that have been expelled from this life stream, or ones from where the stream gets dammed up and congested; wood appears where the plant hardens, nectar appears where growth ends in flower development, sugar in fruits and berries, starch in grains, and fats and oils in embryos and seeds, where growth forces get closed off and terminated in fruits. These substances tend to be fine or less coarse in fully active life processes such as the ones in greening shoots. Green leaves don't contain much sugar, starch or fats. When a plant's etheric processes weaken its essence falls into the physical plane. and "shatters" into matter.

Vitamin B_1 or thiamine becomes detectable wherever starch and sugar accumulates in plants. It helps the organism to get rid of this accumulation of carbohydrates in the right way, and to take hold of the life process when it wants to get started up again in germination and sprouting. There is a lot of Vitamin B_1 in the proteinaceous husks around grain kernels, and their removal by an inevitable grinding process can lead to beriberi and other severe nutritional disorders. This thiamin process is coupled with a phosphorus process or a phosphorylase in the human organism that facilitates a proper degradation of carbohydrates in the brain and muscles. If this oxidation is incomplete one gets accumulations of acid breakdown products, an overloading of the brain and nervous system with succinic acid, of the heart and other muscles with lactic acid, together with brain convulsions and paralysis of muscles; – man's higher members are pushed back by organs that are overloaded with acids.

A lot of vitamin B_1 is produced by the yeasts that stimulate the fermentation of sugars, and by other organisms that have to live on carbohydrates to a large extent.

This is the place to say a few things about the relation of coarse and fine substances to plants' biological processes. Neither group of substances is anything primary, for they both arise out of the life process and out of the nature of the formative forces that interact with earthly matter. The primary thing is the super-physical action of formative forces, and everything that clothes a plant in a sensory, material way arises from the nonmaterial or supersensible sphere. The supersensible life activity and the force form comes first, and the forming and ordering of substances springs from there. However, all of this would not be possible if the earthly world of substances and materials did not provide a point of contact for such efforts.

Lifeless earthly substances belong to the gravitational, cohesive, etc. forces that are bound to the centers of material things and that radiate from them as centrifugal forces, and that form force fields around the centers of material things which quickly get weaker further out and eventually disappear. But earth substances don't just belong to this realm of centrifugal forces, they can gradually strip off their relations to it and open themselves entirely to the completely opposite realm of universal forces that streams in from the world's periphery. The three dimensional, coarse material aspect is mainly connected with the first realm of forces.

If one dimension of this ponderable form of existence is sacrificed, if earth matter goes over into a two dimensional, colloidal existence, and if it thereby becomes materially dispersed, it partly withdraws from earthly, centrifugal forces, opens its doors to cosmic, universal forces and develops relations with them. The organic forces of the biological world and the holistic forces in the etheric bodies of living beings are woven together from the ocean of these universal forces that work in out of the cosmic periphery.

A plant that puts its roots into the coarsely material body of the earth. and opens its leaves to the cosmic environment has connections with both of these kinds of forces. In its ponderable materiality it leans towards earthly forces and is thereby a corporeal, earthly entity. However it has opened its finer materials to the actual life forces and has thereby created instruments with which it can intervene in coarse materiality and control its processes.

If one takes "vitamins" out of their fine material state and concentrates them into a normal, three dimensional, coarsely material condition, they lose their mysterious aspect, and then vitamin C, for instance, has become a white material that looks like salt, i.e., it has become ascorbic acid, or something that has the same value as all the other acids a chemist has in his laboratory. A vitamin is not a vitamin by itself, through its materiality, but only through its connection with the biological activities of an organism, just as a clock pendulum by itself is only a bar with a heavy disk at its end, and it is only a pendulum if it is attached to the rest of the clock. All of the finely material substances that have been discovered in such large numbers since the beginning of the 20th century are materials of the boundary between matter and formative forces, between the physical and etheric worlds, which are therefore suitable for the transmission of the impulses of the etheric body of a live organism to the physical body.

The main functions of the etheric body are to bring about growth, healing, reproduction, etc. and therefore they are faithfully reflected in the hormones, biotic and other fine substances that are connected with growth, healing, reproduction, etc. The antibiotics that can stop and paralyze these biotics are in the same position.

People who have tried to understand how biotics work have given them the capacity to intervene in oxidations and hydrations or reductions as so-called redox systems. No doubt the interaction of the oxygen process with the biological activities or organisms is something that is very important. Rudolf Steiner described the primal, phenomenal role of oxygen with respect to life functions as follows: It draws the etheric organization of an organism down into the physical. This oxygen is an incarnation substance for the etheric in general. It helps to vitalize digested food that has been absorbed by the blood in human organisms. However, this doesn't occur automatically but through the activity of the heart-lung system. (Rudolf Steiner, *Fundamentals of Anthroposophic Medicine*, Oct. 27, 1922). Thus to this extent the idea of biotics as redox systems may be correct for some of them, but such a concept is too one–sidedly chemical.

In Rudolf Steiner's second medical course he pointed out that the chemistry of living things and of lifeless things are just about the opposite; one has to speak of an "anti-chemistry." This indicates that the chemistry of living things is impulsed by an entirely different sphere than ordinary chemistry is. The interplay of universal forces and central ones becomes manifest as the battle of chemistry and anti-chemistry in the organism's transformation of substances.

And in fact a chemist has to learn how to think quite differently when he enters the realm of physiological processes. Everything happens differently here than one is used to in the laboratory. One has to be very much aware of this difference. When process A is led over into process B, a counter wave is set in motion that would like to lead process B back into process A. The organism makes its decisions in the interplay between process and counter process or in the equilibrated events. The transformation of substances goes through a kind of jumping procession; for instance, although the oxidation or disintegration of sugar in muscles to lactic acid occurs with the aid of thiamine and phosphorus, the latter is also converted back to sugar at the same time, except that there are three steps in the direction of disintegration for every two steps in the opposite direction. This is incomprehensible, senseless and impractical from a chemist's point of view. However the important thing for the organism is that its members can exert forces in the transformation of substances, and the latter are inconsequential. An equilibrated physical state must be available for this, and it arises through a meeting of process and counter process.

The Totality of Food Plants

Initially we are nourished by something that is unified and that can let a differentiated organism proceed from it, namely, by our mother's blood before birth, and after birth by the milk that also proceeds from the mother's blood. These and all other foods must be unified in our own blood again before our differentiated organism can be built up out of it.

After infancy our food is a clever combination of things made into a totality in our meals and dishes. Plants and plant parts are prepared and put together by an ordering principle, namely, the "idea of the human organization" as such, that is sometimes grasped consciously but usually instinctively. Edible roots, leaves, flowers and fruits or the whole threefold plant belong to this, because the threefold human organism must be fed. The primal connections between plant and man that are well known to readers of Volume I of this Healing Plants play on important role again here, the head is fed more by potatoes, turnips, carrots and other root foods, the metabolic organism by flowers and fruits, and the rhythmic system by leaves.

This totality of foods is made one-sided in diets, corresponding to the change from the healthy archetype that is brought about by an ailment. Diets are really something like remedies.

Bread is a primal form of human food. The secret of the overall human organization has been taken into it in a many-sided way, and it is active in it. Proper bread must be made out of whole grains. It feeds the entire threefold human being, since the whole threefold plant lives hidden in whole grains and can emerge from them at any time. The individual processes of bread preparation repeat the life process of the grain in its interaction with elements at a higher level with the vital formative forces in the earth's etheric sheath, with "Natura naturans"[15] Just as germinating grain in the ground absorbs fluids, falls apart and sacrifices its life to the shoot, and this opens up to the air in the leaf process, and finally surrender itself to cosmic warmth in the ripening process, so grain is first broken up in the preparation of bread, and its formative forces are ab-

---

[15] People in the Middle Ages used this expression to refer to the creative, developing aspect of Nature which is something supersensible and spiritual, whereas it has been said that the completed side of nature that is accessible to the senses is "Natura naturata."

sorbed in the resulting fine or coarse meal; then the dough is plasticized with the aid of fluids, aerated as it "rises", and finally baked and matured by the heat of an oven. The four membered life processes of a plant in the earth are followed by a fourfold process for making bread in order to serve the four membered human being, with the solid, fluid, airy and warmth organizations that are the housings for one's physical, etheric, astral and I members, as a food that is appropriate for them. If the biological totality of the grain has gone into such a bread, it contains all the necessary vitamins, trace elements, biocatalysts and other things that haven't even been discovered yet, in addition to proteins, carbohydrates and fats—it is actually a totality.

Deficiencies can only arise if food consumption is one-sided. If one strips off the sheath of a fruit one no longer has all the processes through which an inner element comes into interaction with an outer element that builds it up and spurs its development through further growth; the husk and the sheath vitamins that are now called A and B complexes are missing. If one takes away the innermost part of the fruit, the germ, with its fatty oils, one takes away the inner core in which life has contracted so that it can develop again in the outer, phenomenal world. Then one has a deficiency in germ and seedling vitamins D and E, etc. The juice vitamins, like vitamin C are captured in the fluids between the two poles. The husk and the sheath vitamins have a good effect on the region of the skin, senses and nerves, the germ and kernel vitamins have more of an effect on the metabolic region, reproductive processes, etc. Nutrients that have been obtained from healthy plants and that have been built up into a proper, nutritious totality already contain all the necessary biotics and don't need to be supplemented with synthetic vitamins. It is only food that has been prepared from one–sided, injured plants or from ones that have been grown in an unhealthy way that need to be enriched by additives that are obtained from plants that have abnormally intensive processes in their husks and sheathes, or germs and kernels, or juices as in certain wild fruits, etc.

Unfortunately this is often necessary today. Our staple foods have been injured through the way our cultivated plants are being grown by methods that are not in accordance with nature, so that the number of pests is increasing, and one has to combat them with strong chemical poisons that are disguised under the name of plant protecting agents, that not only kill fungi and animal parasites but everything else as well. All these practices of an age that is blind with respect to life make food supplements necessary. One has to be deeply grateful to Nature that she is creatively active in many-sided and one-sided things, and that it has produced things that can cure one sided things when deficient human insight has destroyed the many sided things. One has to be thankful to her that she has one–sidedly created a particularly large amount of vitamins in Sea buckthorn, lemons, rosehips, carrots, nuts, seeds, etc., with which deficiencies can be balanced out.

Summary

The "vitamins" that were discovered in our staple foods at the beginning of the 20th century point to an important biological process through which substances are brought into a fine, material condition in which they are withdrawn from the influence of dead earth forces and are opened up to the vitalizing influence of the etheric cosmic peripheral forces. The etheric bodies of organisms can use substances that stand at the boundary between three dimensional, physical existence and two dimensional, etheric life as mediators and instruments to work into the three dimensional, material world. Thus in principle there are as many vitamins as there are species or as there are etheric processes that work into and control physical substances. Vitamins are tracks which the etheric makes in the physical that deposit from the life stream through a slowing down of etheric processes. Thus, if one takes vitamins or other trace elements out of the physical food substances, organisms that eat such foods can no longer thrive on them. Such substances give rise to metabolic irregularities in organisms.

The author has the pleasant duty of heartily thanking Klaus Jensen, M.D. for the inspiration he gave me for the above section through a paper he wrote for the journal "Beiträge für eine Erweiterung der Heilkunst nach geisteswissenschaftlichen Erkenntnissen" (Contributions towards an Extension of Medicine in Accordance with Spiritual Science Findings)

THE EXTRA-CORPOREAL "ORGANS" OF PLANTS

In Volume I of *Healing Plants* we pointed to primal connections between plants and men that enable one to understand why medicinal plants are capable of healing human diseases. The threefolding of a plant was compared with that of a human body, and this indicated that leaves have an effect on the rhythmic system, roots on the sensory and nervous systems, and flowers and fruits on the action of the limbs and the metabolism.

Additional insights were gained when the members of plants and humans were compared. A look at the overall nature of a plant shows that it consists of a physical body and a life body; a human being has three "sheathes" around his spiritual core or I, the soul (astral) body, life (etheric) body, and physical body. Thus he has four members while a plant has only two.

Plants are also connected with psychical and spiritual elements, but as members that are not incorporated in them; they are extracorporeal soul and spirit spheres that are forever unborn, weave around each plant, and at most touch them, but never draw into them. Thereby they make a plant into a cosmic being that is open to the world, with the power to be upright like a human being but from, outside not from within. Outer contacts or injuries don't hurt the plant's body or arouse pleasure in it. However the soul that weaves around the plant is glad [16] when it experiences the marvelous harmony in the interaction of all the earthly and cosmic forces of its body; and the outer manifestation of this cosmic joy of the soul is the opening of the flowers. That is why flowers speak to our souls in so many different ways and why one can express the most delicate feelings of the soul with a bouquet. This is also the reason why eastern people have developed the art of flower arranging; painters have recorded their ephemeral work for posterity.

Thus a plant is a four-membered being just as humans are, with the restrictions just mentioned. From this one can arrive at other primal relations of these two beings to each other. These become ever clearer if one follows how the supersensible members or spheres of the being take hold of and permeate the materiality of the physical body that is assigned to them. We should remember that fluids are connected with etheric, formative forces, gases are shaped into an airy organization by the astral, soul forces, and that thereby a soul entity can be incorporated, and finally that warm things enable spiritual things with an egoic nature to incarnate. Accordingly, a plant has a solid and fluid organization, but only the be-

---

[16] According to indications by Rudolf Steiner.

ginnings of its own air and warmth organizations, in contrast to the human being who has all four members and four material states.

Nevertheless, the plant kingdom does have the germs of an air and warmth organization, and the astral and I spheres are active on it from outside. That is why one can treat the members of man's being with plant remedies, as we have indicated for certain plants and for whole families like the labiates, umbellifers, cactuses and chenopods, or fiery, airy, watery and saline plants, just to mention a few.

One also has specific plants that are for ailments of the heart, lungs, liver and kidneys; each human organ has one or more plants that mainly work upon it. That seems to be very mysterious at first, since a plant has no inner organs like the ones humans have. So why is it that one plant has a pronounced healing effect on sick hearts and another on the kidneys, etc.? What mysterious connections exist between the plant kingdom and a person's inner organs? This inner world is a real cosmos of organs with wonderfully harmonized connections. This inner cosmos of organs enables each person to give impulses to the body from the center of one's being. Free decisions can activate this body. But now how are things with a plant? All kind of activities are continuously going on in it also. However these are mostly controlled from outside by the weather, times of the day, seasons, the positions of the stars, etc. The decision to lift my arm makes demands upon my organism's carbohydrate metabolism. The only thing in a plant that works like this is something external, namely, the hour and season that is given by the position of the sun. The impulses to move a plant's sap and to control its metabolism come from the gigantic, extra corporeal cosmic sphere that encloses the surface of a plant leaf in an ideal way. What a palpable organ in the human body does from within is carried out in a plant through an extracorporeal influence.

How one has to dare to think what a plant really is, namely, a sensible supersensible entity, which is something that Goethe already knew. One has to think of "extracorporeal plant organs", or of organs that have a function that involves forces but no physical body yet, and therefore no spatial shape or fixation at a particular place in space, as one expects from a bodily, physical plant organ. The sought for extracorporeal plant organs haven't been made physical yet, and one has supra–physical, active formations. One has activities in them but no "realities" in the usual sense.

The big step in the creative world process beyond the plant is that outer spheres of activity are interiorized and they appear as inner organs in animals and humans. This process was realized step by step, as one can see in the "lower" animal kingdom, that has fewer and more primitively shaped organs than the higher animals, but that is connected much more intensively with cosmic events and with the earth processes in its environment, and is somehow "grown together" with them. This "anastomosis" is even greater in plants.

*

A human being also goes through a kind of a plant form of existence at an early, embryonic state of his bodily development, where no inner organs have been formed yet, and all activities flow through the embryonic sheath to the embryo from outside. The whole earth also had an early, embryonic period, for it is a being that is very much alive; it developed out of the maternal sheath of the whole cosmos. The following description of this development is based on the extensive results of Rudolf Steiner's research. [17]

The early forms of the present earth being were strengthened by these sheaths and were fed with things that helped to build them up; the earth floated or swam in a primal atmosphere of fine, fluidic and volatile substance, in a living materiality that one can only compare with present day eggwhite, since it was a substance that was permeated by life. Later on when the earth being condensed, hardened and mineralized, this living, primal atmosphere or biosphere became more rarefied. However, our present atmosphere still contains all the elements that one finds when one destroys eggwhite or other proteins, carbon, oxygen, hydrogen, nitrogen, sulfur, etc.

The mineral, dead earth and its rocks, waters and ocean of air gradually separated from an organic, live primal one, somewhat in the way that a dead, mineralized skeletal system separates from a soft, vital embryonic formation, and remains as a skeleton after death. Thus live, primal protoplasm did not arise from dead hydrogen, nitrogen, etc., through a gigantic "primal synthesis", life came first, and not death. Our

---

[17] Rudolf Steiner, *Occult Science; Mystery Knowledge and Mystery Centers*

present oxygen, nitrogen, etc. "dried out of" live, primal substances, in which formative forces and matter were still firmly united.

A cosmic separation of gigantic proportions had already preceded the earth's development that was just mentioned, for the sun, planets and finally the moon, separated from the undifferentiated, primal world body, and the entire solar system was arranged in an organic way. What had originally been a macrocosmic egg condition with a big mixture of formative forces, realms, creator beings and their shaping impulses, now became a well organized system, each of whose members acquired an individual nature and special function with respect to the whole. A tremendous cosmic formation of organs had thereby taken place. The activities and the special formative forces of the planets, sun and moon now streamed in from outside like organ activities, and permeated the egg-white atmosphere that was mentioned above.

The inner cosmos of organs in each human body is a microscopic copy of this macrocosmic organism. The macrocosmic formative realm has been taken inside, contracted enormously, and given to each human body, so that human beings have a heart as an inner sun, the spleen as an inner Saturn, the liver as an inner Jupiter, a gall bladder as Mars, the lungs as Mercury, the kidneys as Venus and the reproductive organs as Moon.

All of this can only be indicated here, the first comprehensive presentation of it was given by Rudolf Steiner in 1911 in Prague as a cycle of lectures, *An Occult Physiology*.

Each human soul could now incarnate completely in this perfect inner world of organs. (So completely that for a while one could be under the delusion that one's own being was of an entirely corporeal nature.)

Plants were unable to participate in this evolution. Their souls and forces that form organs remained something external to them. They were unable to interiorize and to embody this external element. But it is present in them nevertheless. Plants' soul essence or astrality and the impulses that form something like organs in the earthly sheaths of plants and connect them with the formative forces in the earth's atmosphere, radiate in from our planets, sun and moon. The atmosphere is still filled by forces that form organs, just as it was in that long past "embryonic" time in earth evolution that is called the Lemurian age in spiritual scientific literature. We will go into a few details about this below.

Organic Functions of the Earth's Sheaths with Respect to the Earth's Life

On the basis of indications by Rudolf Steiner, Guenther Wachsmuth described the physical and etheric divisions in the earth's atmosphere in such a way that its organ nature and organismic functions in earth life became manifest (Guenther Wachsmuth, *The Etheric Formative Forces in Cosmos, Earth and Man*).

Rudolf Steiner once called the atmospheric region the earth's belly, and he said that the earth's surface was its diaphragm. One would have to look for the earth's head underground. (*Agriculture Course*, in Koberwitz, Lecture 2, 1924).

If we follow the above descriptions and take a close look at this "abdominal space", we see that it has two main zones, each of which is quite differentiated. However, we're dealing with things that flow into each other in a rhythmic and live way here and not with rigidly separated regions. The main two zones that were mentioned differ in the amount of substances that are present in them, that is, there are more substances in the region near the earth's surface. Solids rise up as dust; fluids go much higher as clouds and fall back down again as rain. The gaseous element spreads out and becomes less and less dense the higher it goes. Finally the space around the earth becomes quite cold as one moves away from the latter but quite high up it begins to get warmer again, and the whole earth becomes enclosed by a mantle of warmth (its existence was spoken of by the above mentioned authors decades before it was discovered by natural scientists).

Metals and other earthy substances are also present in very fine, superhomeopathic doses all the way up into the second sphere.

This second zone is characterized by the withdrawal and disappearance of substances and by the predominance and finally the sole presence of the world of formative forces. The four kinds of ether in the latter also permeate the first zone that is filled with substances, life ether permeates solids, chemical ether fluids, light ether gases and warmth ether permeates warmth. The varieties of ether have close evolutionary connections with the so-called aggregate states of matter. The stepwise condensation of a primal condition of warmth to air, fluids and solids in the course of earth evolution was accompanied by a progressive refinement of warmth ether to light to chemical to life ethers. So in a way the airy element is a "house" for light ether, fluids and water are a house for chemical ether, etc. Thus the ethers permeate the matter in the lower zone with their forces, whereas they are present in their pure etheric form in the upper zone.

This zonal division and layering is subject to the diurnal rhythm and to the life of the earth being, and it is not a rigid thing. These zones stream through each other and combine and separate in the phenomenon of "earth respiration". At dawn the life ether and chemical ether press out from the solid earth in a large exhalation process, while the light and warmth ethers come down in a centripetal way. The first two expand, the latter two press in. The daily variations in barometric pressure, temperature, light intensity, ionization, and in the formation of fog and dew, etc., are an expression of this etheric respiration. Rhythms of the liver, gallbladder and kidneys, etc., run parallel with these rhythms of the earth's sheath that one could call organismic. One can find synchronous and symphonic rhythms in the earth's etheric body and in the human etheric body (G. Wachsmuth). In the twelfth lecture of *Spiritual Science and Medicine* that Rudolf Steiner gave to doctors on April 1, 1920, he said some basic things about the relations of human organs to the atmospheric life that becomes manifest in meteorological events. In the preceding lecture he had said that the gravity of the air in a place works upon the life of the bladder and kidneys. The quality of the warmth upon the heart's action, the quality of water upon liver processes, etc. But on this occasion he pointed to a function of the interaction of these "meteorological organs" that is a completely new discovery and is of great importance. "These four organ systems are nothing less than the creator of the structure of human protein." We must think of the inner constitution of protein "as a result of what proceeds from these four organic systems. Protein is the result of the interaction of these four organ systems. This also tells one something about the interiorization of outer activities in man."

Thus an interiorization of something that otherwise only occurs out in Nature occurs in the formation of human organs with the formation of protein. Steiner says:

"But things are different with vegetable protein. Plant protein is not under the influence of four organ systems, or at least it seems not to be (italicized by the present author), it is under another influence, namely, that of oxygen, nitrogen, hydrogen, carbon and of the sulfur that mediates between the functions of these four. The four substances that are dispersed in the atmosphere bring about the same thing in plant protein that the heart, lungs, liver, etc. bring about in human beings. Extra human Nature contains the same formative forces in these four substances that are present in the four organ systems in intrahuman nature in an individualized way."

The primal connection between the activity of organs and the elements in air that arose through the decomposition of the primal, "albumin atmosphere" and that are interiorized in human organs, exists for plants as something that is outside them. According to this view, the primal, albumin atmosphere was permeated by formative tendencies and vital formative forces that have turned towards the formation of inner organs with their power to shape protein. However, the tendencies and forces that remained outside in the weaving of oxygen, nitrogen, etc. in the atmosphere represent the extra-corporeal organ sphere of plants that creates protein in them. In order to understand this, one has to look at the formative forces that permeate these elements and not just at their dead, material side, which inorganic chemists investigate in their laboratories. One should look at each substance in connection with its field of formative forces. So "when we speak of oxygen, hydrogen, etc., we shouldn't just think of the forces in the substances of which modern chemists speak, we should realize that these substances are endowed with formative forces and powers to act upon things, which always have a relation to each other as their activities increase the store of earthly substances." (All of these quotations are from the lecture Rudolf Steiner gave to doctors on April 1, 1920.)

Rudolf Steiner went on to say, "If we go into the details and we want to equate what oxygen does when it stays outside with inner organs, we would have to identify it with the inner renal–urinary system. We must identify what carbon does when it unfolds its formative forces outwardly with the inner pulmonary system, insofar as the lungs have their own formative forces, and not insofar as the lung system is merely a respiratory system. We must identify nitrogen with the liver system and hydrogen with the heart system. The hydrogen outside is really the heart of the outer world, nitrogen is the liver of the outside world, etc."

Elsewhere Rudolf Steiner spoke even more concretely about forces that form organs and that still permeate the atmosphere today. He said approximately the following about this in the first lecture of September 22, 1922, "Supersensible Influences in the History of Mankind".

Air mainly contains oxygen, nitrogen, carbon dioxide noble gases, sulfur compounds and hydrogen, but it also contains solid minerals and many other materials in an extraordinarily dilute form. In their "normal", solid state these substances have the tendency to form crystals. The highly diluted, fine substances that are in an etheric, super homeopathic or formative force condition also have the tendency to create forms, but these are the forms of human organs and not mineral forms. The air contains fine, etheric formations that correspond to the forms of liver, lungs, etc. These are huge, mighty, etheric formations that permeate the space that surrounds us in the universe. "We can see all human forms in the world ether, if we are trained to see etheric beings." (Lecture of 9/22/22, page 2)

So if the formative forces of inner human organs begin to get weak, there are a lot of healing forces available in the air. The present atmosphere is still filled by the interactions of physical substances, etheric formative forces and impulses that form organs that were mentioned in connection with the albumin atmosphere in past stage of earth evolution. Plants build up the greatest part of their bodies out of the atmosphere, which contains the "extra-corporeal plant organs."

When we look at a human organ we must distinguish between the physical organ and its specific protein substances, the etheric organ and its characteristic constitution of formative forces, the way in which the four kinds of ether interact in it, and the astral part that the overall astral body sends into the organ, and finally the portion that the I-being sends toward the organ. The entire human being is active in every part of his bodily organization and he expresses himself in every detail and organ with his four-membered overall being. Therefore it is important to know how the astral body and I send their impulses into each other, and not just to know how the physical part and its etheric, formative forces are constituted. For instance, in the liver one should note its relatively high temperature and its plastic, fluidic aspect at the physical level, and how its chemical and warmth ethers predominate at the etheric level (its chemical achievements are many). The astral body makes it into an organ that secretes bile. It is a major participant in carbohydrate metabolism, and as such it serves the I-being.

If we look for the extra-corporeal plant organ that corresponds to the liver we must ascribe a physical part, an etheric part and the accompanying astral influences and I impulses to it. As we indicated, atmospheric nitrogen bears the physical part of this "plant liver region". Etheric formative tendencies permeate it, and we have to pay particular attention to the chemical and warmth ethers in it. We noted that there are plenty of gigantic, etheric liver forms in the universe. As we showed in the introductory sections of Volume I, the astral influences and the plants' astral bodies stream in out of the cosmic periphery, and that is from the planets into the earth's atmosphere. One will associate Jupiter with the "liver regions". (The liver is the inner Jupiter in the human organ cosmos.) The plant Is radiate their forces down from the sun and into the physical, etheric, and astral formations we described. They are active in the line between the sun and the earth's center, into which each physical plant with its impulse to stand upright is placed.

Each human *kidney* has mainly developed its physical part into an organ that takes in and secretes fluids. It is also the organ that contains the most *oxygen* and it has something to do with the development of inner light processes. Chemical and light ethers are active in its etheric part in a major and controlling way. A kidney's portion of the human astral body is particularly important, for the kidney process integrates the whole astral body into the metabolic system.

The *physical part of the outer, atmospheric kidney* region of plants must be looked for in the atmosphere's *oxygen*, and the etheric formative forces that belong to it are the *light* and *chemical ethers* that are interacting out there. The corresponding astral impulses radiate in from the Venus sphere, and I impulses come in from the sun.

Likewise, one has to look upon the *carbon processes in the atmosphere* as the *physical, lung organ of a plant being*, and upon the interaction of *life* and *light* ethers as this lung's etheric body; these two ethers have special connections with carbonaceous things. *Mercury's* planetary sphere radiates in the corresponding astral impulses.

This view also says that the atmosphere's *hydrogen* is the plant's physical "heart", and that its etheric heart arises through the interweaving of *life* and *warmth* ethers; its *astral impulses come from the sun*.

Rudolf Steiner also brought out another aspect of the relations of plants to the astral or soul sheath that envelops the earth just as the atmosphere does. Plants stick their flowers into this "soul sheath" of the earth and relate to it through their flowery nature. The earth's astrality becomes specialized with respect to each plant species in a way that is in accordance with its nature. The part of the earth's soul that sinks down into a lily has a different outer aspect than the part that goes into a clover blossom, etc. "The relationship that exists between the whole earth's astrality and the plants that cover the earth also exists inwardly between the human astral body and its individual organs." (GA 156, 12/13/14) This relation between plants and man's inner organs also becomes manifest in something else, namely, in the specific ability of each organ to smell the plants that belong to it. "It is really true, and I'm not just speaking symbolically, when I say that a particular plant that grows outside can only be tasted by a particular organ in human beings, and other organs cannot taste it. One particular organ permits itself to be stimulated by the forces of a particular plant. Once one studies these connections one will know something that is very important." (Ibid). Remedies made from particular plants enable one to bring their specific relationship to the earth's astral sphere into human beings, and this is a healthy relationship. If there is an unhealthy relation between the human astral body and an organ, and if this organ's ability to taste things has become dull, the forces of a particular plant will remedy this astral deficiency.

Rudolf Steiner concluded that one will be able to set up a new, rational system of medicinal plants by finding the correspondence between human organ forces and the forces of plants. He laid the foundation for such a botany in the statements we quoted.

THE NITROGEN, OXYGEN, CARBON AND HYDROGEN ORGANS IN THE ATMOSPHERE

Nitrogen

We already mentioned that Rudolf Steiner said that in some respects nitrogen is the "outer world's liver". In order to understand such a statement one should recall what the main function of this organ is. The human liver receives food from the outside world that has been digested in the outer tract, and acts as a "chemicator" of the body – a chemist and a chemistry laboratory at the same time. It leads food over into the processes that build up the body. This vital chemistry of the body takes place in a particularly warm region; the organ that is chemically the most active is also the warmest one. The chemical ether and warmth ether are the main forces in the liver's etheric body.

The liver also separates off a bile process, whereby iron is expelled from the blood and the coloring matter in the bile is formed.

We now want to take a look at a spherical sheath or zone around the earth about 45-60 miles up in the air. The radiations and forces from the entire cosmic periphery press into it from outside. They cannot be permitted to press down in an unchanged form, they must be digested and assimilated. The earth is like a gigantic organism that is being fed fine substances and force impulses by the universe, and that is giving substances and forces back again. The northern lights that shine at this height have a distinct green, nitrogen line in their spectrum, so that there must be a lot of nitrogen there. It is known that the composition of the atmosphere changes as one goes higher. The lighter elements increase, and the nitrogen that already is 80% of the atmosphere near the earth becomes almost all of it in this higher zone. Physicists estimated that the temperature up there was about $100°C$, and American and Russian rockets and measuring stations later confirmed this. Rudolf Steiner had already spoken about a warmth mantle of the earth already years before the physicists did. This region corresponds to the second, predominantly etheric zone in the earth's sheath that we mentioned earlier, and chemical ether is more active than the other ethers here. We should mention another interesting occurrence in the region. This is where the most meteors and shooting stars lighten up, as the product of an iron process is excreted. The iron is very fine and more functional than material; a very fine dust consisting of meteoric iron falls down slowly. In rare cases a large pile of stone or iron gets through from that sphere. However, the light that radiates in from the cosmos still has the full ultraviolet radiation that is so chemically potent. Thus we have a mighty, physical nitrogen organ before us in which warmth and chemical forces interact, from which an iron process is continually being excreted, and which therefore bears the basic elements of liver dynamics in it.

Oxygen

Another atmospheric earth organ forms out of the air's oxygen process. Oxygen is generated by cosmic light forces and it rises from the founts of life in green plants; it is the universal breathing element near the earth. However it changes its form in the highest strata of the ocean of air. First it becomes more and more rarefied, but at about a height of 15-20 miles, it turns into something quite different under the influence of a light that is becoming ever more cosmic. The oxygen of the lower levels condense into ozone and forms a layer around the whole earth. Thereby it filters out some of the light force that would work upon the organisms on earth in an overly strong and lethal way. This ozone organ of the earth determines which kinds of light can come out of the upper earth sheaths and into the biological layer at the bottom of the ocean of air, with its plants, animals and human beings. An amount of ultraviolet radiation that promotes life is let through and the rest of the rays that belong to this chemical ether are stopped, for they would destroy all life on earth. A great deal in earth life depends on this regulation process, as for instance the pigmentation process in humans and animals, and the formation of the vitamin D that is essential for healthy bones. Thus the earth's oxygen organ is active between the light and chemical ethers. The yellow rays and other elements in light near the ground form oxygen via the green pigments in leaves. The light in the heights converts it to ozone. The more it rays down the more ozone it forms, which thereby blocks off its further course down to the earth. Oxygen therefore is born from light, formed by light and transformed by light. This region also includes the sphere of meteorological events, cloud formations, rainfall and the drawing up of water into the atmosphere again.

Let's take a look at the renal and adrenal process in the human being. Kidneys consume more oxygen than any other organ. The astral organization that ensouls all air processes in human beings inserts itself in the latter through the kidneys. People with kidney diseases have trouble with their breathing. Watery fluids arise through the kidney's activity, are attracted by the bladder's air space and are partly excreted, but a large part of this water is immediately reabsorbed. A healthy color of the skin depends upon the adrenal process. Rudolf Steiner was the first to point out that the kidney process has another task in the organism. It serves the development of an inner light, the generation of "primal light". Our system has yet to get enough inner light. (see Rudolf Steiner's *Spiritual Science and Medicine*, lecture 11, for more details.)

Thus the interweaving of light and chemical ethers and of the activities of air and water is characteristic for both the kidney and oxygen processes.

Carbon

Carbon is the "lungs of the outer world" according to the view we are presenting here. What is characteristic about its "functionality" in the whole earth process? Does it have an organ function in the life of the whole earth? Just as oxygen shows its nature in an interaction between gases and liquids, and light and chemical ethers, carbon does so in an interplay between aeriform and solid things, and between light and life ethers. It becomes an atmospheric element when it combines with oxygen, and this becomes a carbohydrate in the rhythmic plant organs under the influence of light, and from there it can solidify into wood and become coal. If it is attracted by calcareous elements in the earth it can become solid limestone, dolomite or spar. It is led out of the solid bodies of men and animals into the atmosphere again by their rhythmic respiratory organs. For animals and men do not permit the carbon in them to become as stiff and solid as plant carbon. Carbon becomes deposited along with iron in the tremendous coal belt that runs parallel to the mighty iron belt through the middle of the northern temperate zone, around the whole earth where one has the most dry land. Dissolved in water, it gets into the earth's water cycle. The carbon process helps to regulate the earth's whole oxygen process. It fetters the latter when it combines with elements in the air, or it liberates oxygen and deposits as solid carbon. The carbon process that surrounds a plant takes the place of its missing lung organ. If one were to imagine that the airy environment of a tree was filled with living protein that is shaped and structured by atmospheric forces, which inhales the oxygen that is generated by the tree and exhales carbon dioxide towards it, and if one made the tree invisible and the environment visible, one would have a pulmonary formation, with a bronchial surface and air tubes, or the whole "bronchial tree". However this "external lung" of the plant remains a purely etheric formation that consists entirely of forces.

Hydrogen

Hydrogen is the lightest earthly substance and it strives up to the uppermost regions of the earth's sheath. It would also like to give levity forces to whatever it take hold of and to take it away from gravity. When it combines with oxygen it gives itself some weight again and becomes dense water. The expressions of hydrogen's essential nature fluctuate between lightness and heaviness in this way.

One of hydrogen's main features is its relation to warmth; one can look upon it as a projection of warmth into the world of substances. Warmth has two sides to its nature, it can unite with earthly substances as if it were a substance and be conducted from one body to another and help to determine the form and solidity of substances. On the other hand it can weave through space as radiant warmth, like light, weightlessly and independently of bodies. Solar and terrestrial events and the worlds of cosmic levity and earthly gravity meet in warmth. The closest to it of all earthly substances is hydrogen. One can see this from all of its properties. Hydrogen is the governor of warmth in the realm of substances. It is warmth that has a minimum of matter attached to it. As it combines with other earthly substances it wants to desolidify and lighten them and carry them back to the region of pure warmth in the cosmos. Therewith it wants to give them back to the creative chaos that was the primal and starting condition of earth evolution, its seed condition and beginning, back in the warmth cosmos of "Old Saturn".[18] One gets more and more hydrogen compounds in plants the closer one gets to flower and seed formation; they absorb intense, cosmic, warmth forces as they are formed. The etheric and fatty oils should be mentioned here. A plant's hydrogen process drives it towards the formation of seeds and into a material chaos where the seed's protein strips off all earth forces and opens itself entirely to the cosmos which doesn't just ray down ripening warmth but formative, real, archetypal pictures carried by warmth that make the seed cell into an embryo, and make a new development and next year's life possible. However, just as a ray of warmth enters a substance and warms it, so the seed that is created by the cosmos turns away from the warmth realm again and goes into the realm of gravity and earthly forces. The seed falls down and belongs to the earth again.

One can find what occurs in a plant on a seemingly small scale in a hydrogen process between gravity and levity, and terrestrial and cosmic realms on a gigantic scale in the water life of the whole earth. The evaporating water that has been taken hold of by warmth rises like a gigantic world plant from the earth into cosmic heights, borne up by levity forces. It displays a change in form in the region of cloud formation

---

[18] See R. Steiner, *Occult Science, an Outline* (chapter about world evolution).

with its plastic forms, which is also present in the metamorphosis of leaves in a somewhat different way. The plastic, round and swelling lower leaves correspond to stratus and cumulus cloud formations in the lower atmosphere. And just as the upper leaves in a plant become ever finer and more divided and feathery, so cirrus or feather clouds form higher up in the sky. The cloud being ascends into the cosmic regions that are its flowering sphere, blooms in lightning storms and feeds on fertilizing, cosmic forces. Then comes the dramatic turning point. Rain is formed and plunges to the earth in a million drops as a fertilizing fall of seeds from this gigantic water plant. This is a primal event in which the water that permeates countless plants as a living element can be a plant itself and can rise from microcosmic to macrocosmic regions. That is how Rudolf Steiner once explained it to the workers on the Goetheanum building.

The human heart is an organ that lives in harmony between levity and gravity in many respects. This is indicated by the place it occupies in the body. The two poles between which the heart is active rhythmically are the head organization that stands above it, and opens itself to the light through the senses, is farthest removed from the earth and its gravity, removes the brain from gravity almost entirely, and reflects the cosmic sphere in its curvature and roundness. The metabolic limb system lives under the heart with its pair of columns or legs that are inserted into the lines of gravity and the metabolism that takes earthly substances into it. The heart process is connected to the warmth system through the blood's warmth, so that it is also a harmonizing organ in this respect; for the mean temperature of 98.6% between the hotter arterial blood and the cooler venous one is precisely maintained in the heart. The blood process moves from the body into the heart as if into its innermost core or into a seed condition, comes to rest there for a moment, dies in its movement, and sprays out into the periphery again and goes through a continual dying and becoming with every heartbeat. Thus one can perceive the activities of the warmth and life ethers in the heart process. Organic processes of expansion and condensation are impulsed by the polar exertions of force of these two kinds of formative forces.[19]

---

[19] See Guenther Wachsmuth, *The Etheric Formative Forces in Cosmos, Earth and Man.*

A plant has no inner organ that corresponds to our heart, but it too unfolds its whole being between cosmic levity and earthly gravity. It streams its formative power out into the periphery and pulls it together again in seed formation; this is a real pulsation, but it is stimulated and controlled from outside by the sun forces in the world. However, the fact that the physical substances of a plant can follow this pulsing biological rhythm is only made possible by the way hydrogen is constituted and by the way it bears lightness into heaviness, and the cosmic into the terrestrial sphere.

Some people think that they have discovered a major solar process in the tremendous radiant energies that are liberated on the sun in the transformation of hydrogen. No doubt our ideas about life on the sun are still much too earthly and materialistic. (Some people even think that they'll be able to imitate the solar process on earth by transforming hydrogen into helium.) In any case, the hydrogen process that surrounds us everywhere on the earth is a mighty connective process between earthly and cosmic beings that is turned towards solar forces and not just towards terrestrial ones. Earthly matter is extended to something solar by hydrogen and it opens up a path for solar forces into nature on earth.

A plant has no inner heart, but because it has hydrogen it is attached to external world processes that represent its heart action.

The following eight pictures that were made by H. Krüger in accordance with E. Pfeiffer's sensitive copper chloride crystallization method and that were kindly put at our disposal, tell us something about the relation of certain medicinal plants to forces that form organs. What we have here are four pictures of copper chloride crystallizations that were made by adding very small amounts of juice from an animal heart, lung, liver and kidney to copper salt solutions, which were then allowed to crystallize slowly. Each of these pictures has forms that are characteristic for the particular organ. Four other pictures were placed alongside these that were obtained in the same way, except that juices from medicinal plants that are known to cure diseases of these particular organs were put into the solutions, rather than animal organ juices. The pictures speak for themselves (and need no further commentary).

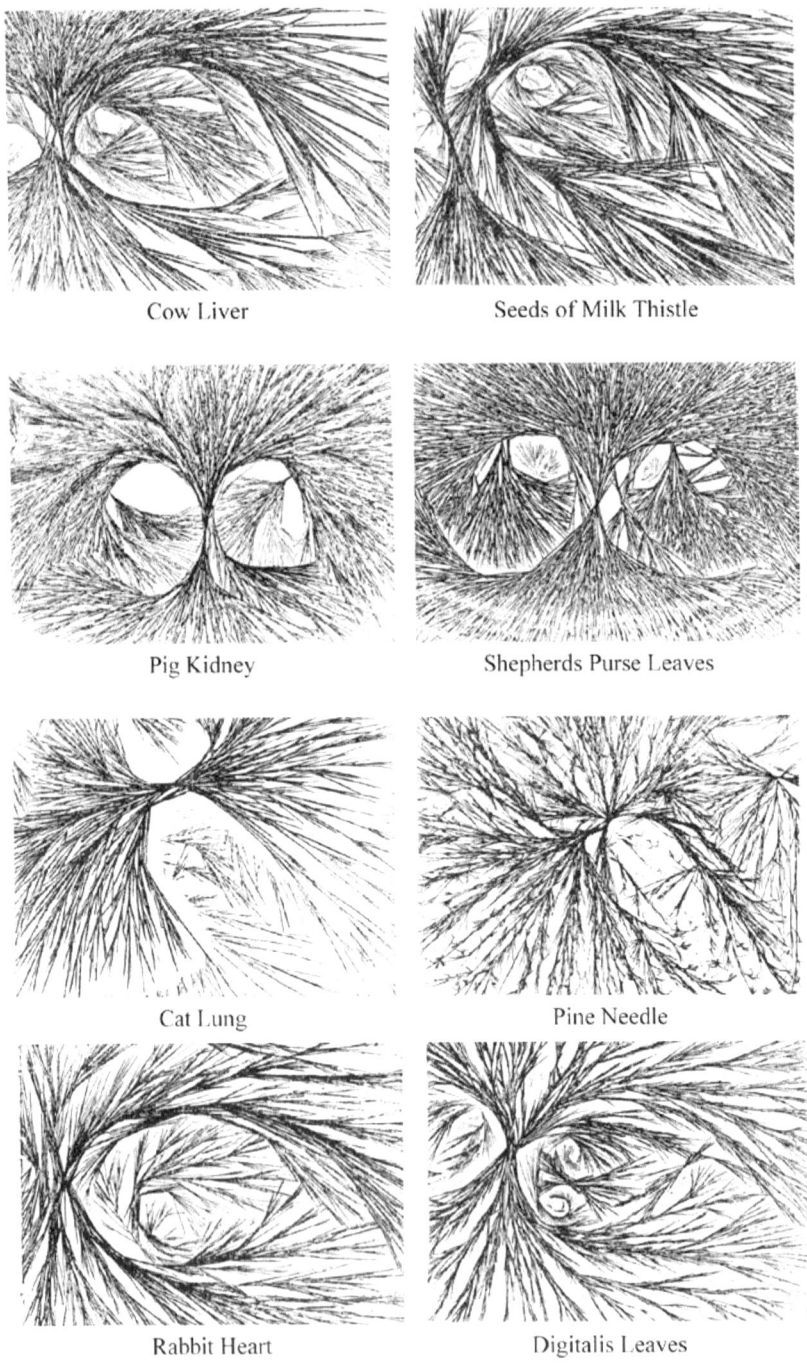

Myrtles – Myrtaceae
Fruit and Spice Plants

There are over 2800 species of myrtles, which makes them one of the large families in the plant kingdom. They can be compared with the rose family in some respects, not from the viewpoint of a botanical systematics, but from one that looks at processes. Both families have an overly strong sugar process, and myrtles are the second largest fruit family after roses. However, unlike the rose family, fruits and other plants that typically inhabit the northern temperate zone, myrtles belong to the tropics of all continents. There are a few myrtle shrubs in the temperate zones, but otherwise they are trees which often have very hard woods.

Myrtle trees oppose sparse, strictly ordered forms to the mighty, proliferating forces of earth and water and to the tremendous warmth influences of the tropics; they tame the rampant tropical forces. Their leaves are evergreen, leathery and smooth edged or sometimes they are contracted into needles. The myrtaceas have strong flowering processes and scents which they open up to animals. Insects and birds are the pollinators. The flower petals can be fleshy or can become a sweet confection. As in the rose family, they surround a large number of stamens; the fruits are usually leather skinned berries or capsules, which form under the receptacle as in the roses. The tropical warmth processes ripen sweet fruits such as varieties of guavas, the cranberry-like fruits of myrtle bushes in the Andes, hill gooseberry, strawberry guava, the sloe-like jambul fruits, rose apple, Brazil cherry, Surinam cherry, Jambolam plum and many others. But they also permeate leaves, flowers, wood and bark and they generate essential oils and aromatic resins. That is why this family has many species. One should mention the aromatic bark of the cinnamon tree (Eugenia caryophyllata), the flower buds of syzygeum aromaticum (spice cloves), the smell of myrtle flowers, allspice or the powdered unripe fruit of the little Pimento tree, the leaf oils of various species of eucalyptus that smell like lemons and peppermint, and the salutary cajeput oil. The myrtles have more strong warmth processes than the rosaceae do, for the latter are matured by moderate warmth in the temperate zones.

After what we said about tannins in the roses and other plants, it will seem incomprehensible that a family that takes in astral forces so intensively through its active flowering process also tends to form a lot of tannins. One could mention the mallee bark of Eucalyptus occidentalis oils here. However, the astral sphere never overpowers the etheric formative forces; there is always a nice equilibrium between the two force realms. That is why myrtles look so harmonious and noble. There are also a few decorative plants among them. And it is right that bridal wreaths are decorated with myrtle flowers. Through the harmony between the polar forces one can also predict correctly that this family produces no poisonous plants; its healthy relations to the earth element become manifest in the production of excellent woods.

The fact that the strong connections of this family to sugar and warmth processes give rise to a species, syzygium jambolana, whose seeds were recommended against diabetes, also reminds one of similar processes in the rose family.

Eucalyptus globulus – Blue Gum Tree, Fever Tree

The myrtle type produces about 160 eucalyptus species under the peculiar climatic and formative conditions of the Australian continent, that have a strong influence on the way landscape looks in this dry and very old part of the earth. This transformative power can be seen in the tall, melancholic eucalyptus forests in the damper southeast, the park trees in the grassy landscapes, the Machialike impenetrable thorn bushes of the dry interior, and in the scrubby bushes on the mountains. A. Usteri, the master of the anthroposophic botanists, says the following about eucalyptus in his *Pflanzensammlung*, (Collection of Plants); "It fits into Australia's uniform vegetation quite well. It belongs together with the dark green Casuarinas. It fits in with the blue green forests of acacia shrub that often extend for miles to the despair of travelers, and with the porcupine grass that creeps along with runners that are many yards long while its prickly, spherical fruits are a plaything for the wind. Eucalyptus is the gloomiest plant among this sorry crowd. It is the melancholic among trees."

Eucalyptus globulus can become a very tall tree that puts its roots deep down into the ground; it knows how to open up the hidden, subterranean water channels in its growing places, and it sucks up all the surrounding water around with great force. If enough of them are planted in a marsh they will quickly lower the water level and remove breeding places for malarial mosquitoes. They grow surprisingly quickly, but still manage to produce a very hard wood with a lot of tannin in it, which therefore decomposes slowly. The active carbo‑ 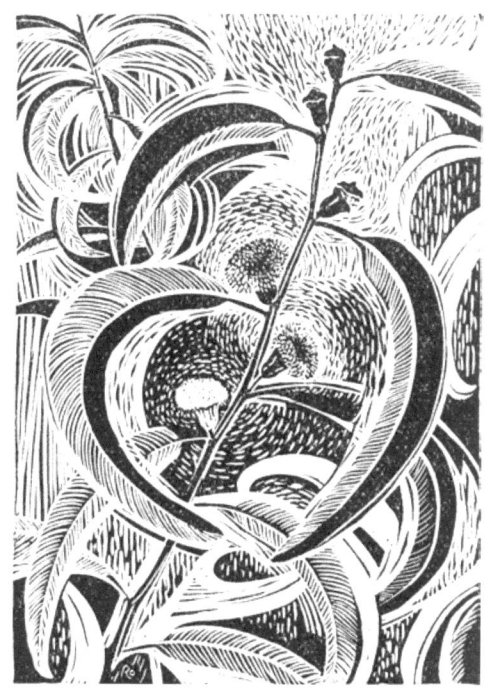 hydrate process in myrtle that leads to burgeoning fruit formation in the dripping tropics becomes converted into the production of wood. Myrtles lignify completely in dry and hot Australian landscapes, right up to the blossoms, where buds look like little handmade wooden boxes that are coated with whitish blue wax and whose petals are shed as a one piece wooden cover as soon as they open; it is pushed off by a large number of stamens that emerge from a boxlike housing that has an ovary that is inserted deep down in the sprouting axil's wooden flowers – what a paradox! Nevertheless, at least part of the sugar process becomes manifest as a source of much nectar at the edge of the inferior ovary, or it can flow out of injured trunks like manna. So there is a myrtle being there, but it is very hardened and lignified. The behavior of its leaf process towards light is also rather peculiar. A young tree has opposite, horizontally placed and seated leaves; however in an older tree the alternate leaves are much longer, narrow and they grow a short petiole that turns itself and the blade by 90 degrees, so that now the leaf's surface is perpendicular, an unusual position that one otherwise only finds in plants that do not want to expose themselves very much to light. One can see from the further developments that above and below, right and left mean something different for a leaf thus positioned; it becomes curved like a sickle, because the upper half of the blade now grows faster and becomes wider than the lower half. Also the two sides of the leaf's surface are anatomically the same, whereas otherwise the upper side is quite different from the underside that is more in the shade. Trees with such leaves let the light flow down to the ground unhindered, and so there is no refreshing shade in an eucalyptus forest. However the dry warmth gives the leathery leaves a mighty etheric oil process that aromatizes the whole tree.

Eucalyptus energetically bears consolidating earth forces and the watery element that is hidden in the depths up into a hot and dry, luminous air region. It attracts the realm of astral beings through an active development of the tannin process, permits the sun's I power that forms essential oils to become very active along a long vertical line and it deals rather circumspectly with the light process in its leaves, which thereby presses into the unshaded depths, all the way down to the root region. The lignification of the carbohydrate process by the earth's forces right into the flower region, or the pushing through of root forces right into the flowers, meets the other tendency to inflame and to form ethereal oils, that is connected with cosmic light processes that are usually reserved for the flower region but that have pressed down into the leaf region here. They let the light go through to where the trunk meets the roots. Both of these push through each other. When we investigate the suitability of this plant to be a remedy, we should be aware of this abnormality in the interaction of life and light.

If the "carbon organ" or lung that is connected with the forces of the earth's configuration[20] surrenders itself too strongly to the influences of the outer world, like a sense organ, external cold and other things can press into it like foreign bodies. The organism responds to this with inflammations and mucous formation. Extracts from eucalyptus leaves or eucalyptus oil are helpful here. In addition one has to keep in mind that ethereal oils have a strengthening effect on the I organization in general, which we discussed in the section about labiates in Volume I.

---

[20] For instance, Rudolf Steiner pointed to such connections in the eight lectures given around Easter 1921. One also knows that certain landscapes with particular soil constitutions make lung diseases worse or better and this is intensified if it is accompanied by certain light conditions.

Eugenia caryophyllata (syzygium aromaticum) – Clove Tree

The clove tree is a real child of the tropical Asiatic Isles and it is comparable to our pear trees in size and growth. Its branches have more of a tendency to bend. The leaves are coarse, leathery, evergreen and in opposition to the triply threefolded inflorescences bear nail shaped, fleshy, cartilaginous, red flowers that bring forth four small sepal. Above them the hood–like petals grown together into a flat cowl over a large number of stamens on the thickened twig that has taken the hypogynous ovary into itself at its upper end. This hood is thrown off at flowering time. However the flower buds are picked or knocked off before this occurs, dried in the shade and sold as cloves. Each tree produces large quantities of them. The glands that are imbedded in the flowers are full of etheric oil that is denser than water, not very volatile, with a pungent aroma. This shows that the cosmic fire forces that generate it have been drawn mightily into the earth region and have become earth–like. The root-earth forces thrust into the flower region in this tree. Gravity is combined with levity in the caryophyllaceous scent. This peculiar earth fire process is combined with something else in the formation of cloves, a formation of a lot of tannin. The astral sphere becomes active in a substance forming way in the formation of tannins, just as this happens with the plant's cosmic I sphere in the formation of etheric oils. Both of these combine and form substances in this plant's flower region.

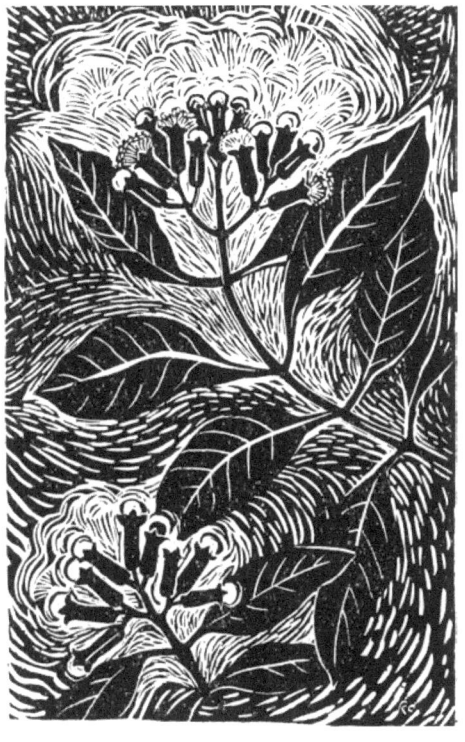

The clove is a pure flower drug, which results in strong effects in the metabolic region – as we saw in the introductory sections of Volume I on threefolded plants and human beings. This spice strengthens one's digestive power against heavy, earthy food in the regions where the breakdown of the latter must be carried out by one's I and astral body, so that it can pass over into individual parts of the body and build them up. Cloves help to regulate digestion. If the latter tends to become too hard so that one has to induce elimination with laxatives, adding some cloves will help this to occur in accordance with the I and astral organizations. In anthroposophic therapy, cloves are included in compound preparations recommended by Rudolf Steiner.

CRANE BILLS – GERANIACEAE

One can get a good idea about what this family is really like by looking at our balcony geranium, Pelargonium zonale, that indestructible decoration of our cities in the summer, which stretches its fleshy leaves with their brownish violet stripes towards the sun and holds up its many dark red flowers on their thick, slimy stems in spite of the glowing heat of the artificial stone deserts and meager water supply. It is basically a fat, congested plant that holds its watery constituents together in an almost succulent way that responds to the broiling summer sun by developing strong and pungent scents in the leaves and by becoming "overdone" in its flowers. Pelargonium can feel uncomfortable in the stone deserts of large cities, because it is a native of Africa's rocky, dry landscape down on the cape. The related Bushman's candle (Sarcocaulon) with its trailing, swollen stems and thorny leaves looks something like a cactus; its scent formation passes over into the formation of a resin that completely covers the puffy stems. Warmer, damper climates produce species with thinner leaves, deep indentations and pinnaform lobes that open themselves up more to the airy element with ennobled aromas that smell like lemons or even roses, and they induce people in Spain, Algeria and on the Reunion and Bourbon islands to grow large numbers of pelargoniums.

One can see the tendency to carry the flowering aspect into a lower region in the fact that their nectaries are on the flower stems.

The over 200 species of pelargonium live mainly in hot and dry South Africa, whereas the over 70 kinds of crane bills prefer the Mediterranean regions. Finally the 260 or so species of geranium are wide leafed plants with nice flowers that belong to the damper, temperate zones; they are sensitive to the distribution of moisture in land and their various species grow accordingly on meadows, dry fields, rocky hills, dumps, at the edges of woods, along rivers and in the shadow of bushes. Here there is no more formation of essential oils in the leaves, but the intensity of the flowering process can be seen in the short life of individual flowers, which drop their petals soon after they open. Bluish and reddish blue shades in the flowers predominate in these "damper" Geraniaceae and they contain quite a few tannins.

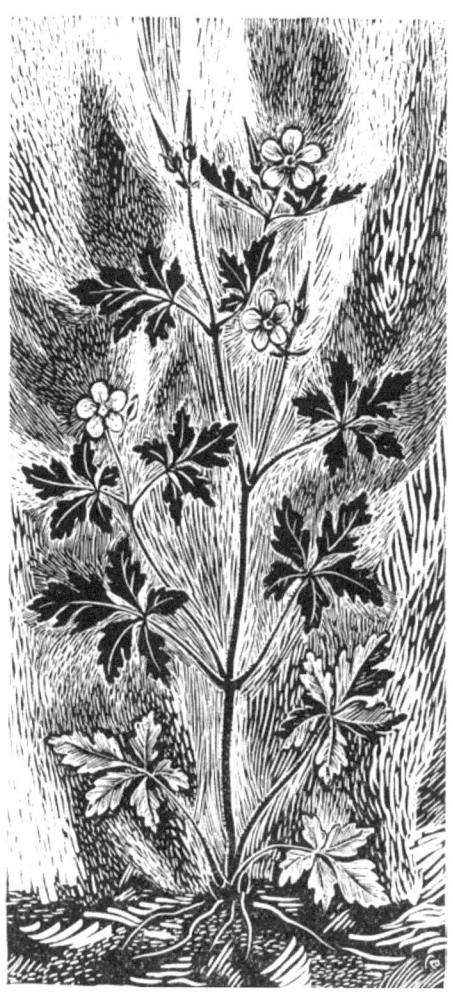

The dry, capsule-like, long beaked fruits (which gave the family its name) are sensitive to the amount of moisture in the air. Depending on the latter, the beak part rolls spirally in and out and when it falls off it bores the fruits and seeds into the earth. People have made simple humidity gauges on the basis of this behavior. Other species hurl their seeds somewhat like touch–me–not does, when the capsules are ripe and dry. This family doesn't form any trees but only herbs which develop in too luxuriant a way to let the strongly attracted warmth forces develop in as fiery a manner as this is possible in labiates, for instance. It can produce aromatic, refreshing substances that smell like lemons or even roses (although a dull, earthy element is not overcome), but it can't compare with the noble fire of a lavender or a rosemary. The dessicated fruit process that is left behind after the flowers have withered remain sensitive to moisture in the air.

In a case where there were peripheral, inflammatory symptoms and tiredness in the limbs, Rudolf Steiner recommended the oral administration of cranesbill that had been roasted and made into a fairly concentrated lactose trituration. A good species to use here would no doubt be Herb Robert, Geranium roberticum, that likes to grow in forest clearings, at the edges of woods, on piles of stones and in hot, waste areas; it has reddish stems and nodes, palmately divided leaves with deeply indented sections that are hairy and sticky, pink flowers striped with darker pink, and "crane's bill" fruits that stick far out of the inflated calyxes. This old medicinal plant almost looks like an emerging inflammation, and the burnt smell of its crushed leaves reinforce this impression. The warmth forces that intervene strongly in the leaf and stem region are at work here. They are enhanced by the roasting process that expels fluids from the plant and tends to aromatize and sublimate the remaining solids. Such a preparation gets the organism to develop its warmth processes at the right place and in a centripetal way, so they don't shoot out into the periphery.

*

Wood Sorrels – Oxalidaceae

The Oxalic Acid Process in Plant and Man

A normal plant form arises through a rhythmic change in the activities of polar formative forces, namely, contracting and expanding. Condensed in a seed, a plant germinates and expands into a shoot, draws together in a node, expands into a leaf, becomes constricted in a calyx, opens up into a flower, contracts into a seed again and swells up into a fruit.

Goethe was the real discoverer of the laws which govern plant life, and he called this normal succession of rhythmical events a regular or progressive metamorphosis that is peculiar to archetypal plants. Through his study of so-called "monstrosities" in the plant kingdom he discovered irregular or retrogressive metamorphosis. His genial observation of Nature permitted him to find the point in such abnormalities where an active principle that is normally concealed because it is mingled with other forces becomes directly visible, and it is not as if the forces of nature had gone haywire there. A proliferated rose or pink is not a mad trick of nature but a revelation of formative forces in a flower that are otherwise toned down by the counter action of a particular sphere, and that work in an undampened manner at their normal place in the shoot and leaf region. Such monstrosities arise because the beings in the astral realm are working too weakly against the vital growth forces or etheric formative forces, whereas they produce a proper flowering process when they are working at their normal intensity. Abnormal formations draw one's attention to this.

Whole plant families can be involved in such progressive or hyper progressive metamorphoses or can be characterized by such a principle, and not just individual plants. One can understand that the shape of a cactus by telling oneself that such a plant gets to the formation of a shoot, but that it holds back all further expansion into branches and leaves in its body and only develops the germs of a separation. One can see something similar in succulent plants in families such as spurges, stone crops, lilies, fig marigolds and stapelia. The dammed up and thereby particularly strong vitality of such plants enables them to live in deserts and other dry regions. The flowering process in such plants is often very imperfect or belated. It can take quite a few years for a cactus or an aloe to bloom.

"Accidental" metamorphoses can show the influence of higher spheres or nonincorporated members upon plants in a different way. A study of plant galls, a kind of "monstrosity", can lead one to an insight into the normal but deeply hidden connections of a higher super-phytic realm of beings to plants. A plant's formative forces are directed into channels that they would not enter by themselves through the stings, depositing of eggs and injection of poisons by gall wasps and flies and through other interventions from outside (hence "accidental" metamorphoses) into various parts of the plant. This gives rise to the strange colors and forms of gall formations like fruits, which have an animal and not a plant origin. To take two examples out of thousands, fruits like cherries grow out of oaks and sages which the plants would never have produced by themselves (sage galls are even edible). Our sweet, edible figs are produced by the stings of gall wasps. Here the higher realm that is connected with an animal being is obviously helping the vegetative plants to metamorphose into something higher. Its relation to the upper pole of plant metamorphosis, flowers and fruit in general becomes clear. A contact between the essences of the lower plant and the higher animal kingdoms takes place here. One can already see this from the great variety of relations of flowers to "their" bats, bees, birds, bumble bees, butterflies, gnats, flies, snails and other animals. But what makes the animal kingdom the higher one? The fact is that it has a higher principle living in it, the soul essence, or an astral body that an animal has in addition to the members of a plant's being. Plant galls and adaptations of flowers to animal forms are only special cases of a much more general and comprehensive, fundamental connection between etheric formative forces and the astral or soul realm in the universe. These connections bring about plants' normal flowering and fruiting processes. When a plant jumps into its upper metamorphosis, its etheric nature can be determined not only by animals with individual souls, but by the entire soul or astral realm of beings – even if it is only from outside.

There are one–sided forms of the kind of metamorphosis that is determined from the astral sphere, just as the succulents develop one sided, etheric characteristics. Hyperastralized families of plants, such as legumes, can be compared with etherically congested ones. We already gave an extensive description of the former in Volume I, but in general they are delicate plants with leaves divided into feathers and smaller feathers, and numerous flowers that smell sweet and voluptuous and have strong and beautiful colors, and often look like butterflies. The flowering process with its formation of colors and scents can also take hold of the leaves, wood and roots; bees and ants are attracted, or they are even given a home. The flowers are very sensitive to terrestrial, cosmic rhythms, and so are the leaves, as one can see in the day and night movements, light and dark positions, rhythmic swinging of the leaves in accordance with the temperature, and even in the reaction to touch. The hyper-etherized succulents are the polar opposite of the hyper-astralized legumes.

Now, there is one family of plants that is placed between these two poles in a wonderful and harmonious way, that leads from one pole to the other, and in which we see a tendency towards succulent congestion as well as one towards intensive astralization. It begins as a kind of a stone crop and ends up something like a clover. For instance, our wood sorrel, Oxalis acetosella, first grows a rhizome that covers itself with fleshy, thickened scales, and it looks something like a shoot on wall pepper, sedum acre. However, this rhizome keeps all the stem and shoot formation to itself; the long stemmed leaves and flowers grow directly out of the ground. Non-European species of oxalis show this even more plainly, they let the root become fleshy or let it swell into bulbs and tubers (O. deppei, O. crassicaulis, O. esailenta). The succulent congestion can also drive up fleshy leaf petals, or it can swell up their bases (O. rusciformis). If the bulb formation is pushed up into the leaf region, it can appear as little offshoot bulbs, and even press up into the flower region (O. brasiliensis). Reproduction by runners, offshoot bulbs, etc. is more common in such plants than by seeds. 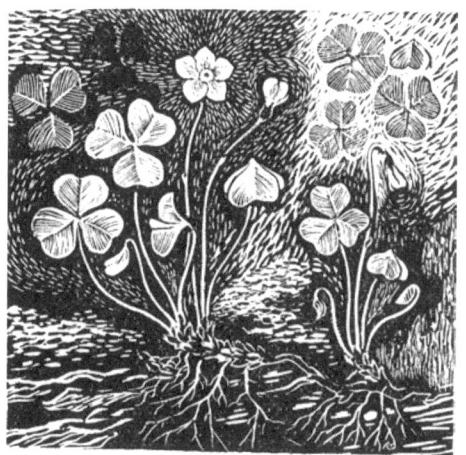 Wood sorrel is one of the species that likes to reproduce via runners. A vegetative activity in some of its flowers takes the place of the normal, astrally conditioned one; it produces hanging flower buds that never open (in addition to normal ones), and the pollen in their anthers grows into the stigmas. Here an etheric process or a vegetative activity replaces the activities of insects or astrally conditioned animals that normally bring pollen to the stigmas.

Thus there is a tendency in the lower organs of wood sorrels to want to become succulent, etherically congested, sedum-type plants, and this even carries over into the flowers. However, the delicate, green, three to ten leaflets per leaf or even pinnately divided leaves withdraw from this congestion; an opposite formative principle becomes manifest in the upper part of the plant. What began as a kind of stone crop like plant seems to want to become a legume. The leaflets in our tripartite, cloverlike wood sorrel leaves are spread out flat in fair weather, and they fold together and hang down during dark and damp weather. The leaves of other species made day and night movements similar to those of beans and locust trees. Biophytum sensitivum is sensitive to touch just like the well known sensitive plant, Mimosa pudica. Oxalis hedysaroides even moves its leaves continuously in slow, jerkily swinging circular rhythms in their tips, something like the legume, Desmodium gyrans. Thus there are similarities between the leaf processes of wood sorrels and those of the pea family, which are not attained by any other plants.

On the other hand, the five petalled flowers are not like those on legumes at all. They have a delicate ray structure and they are brightly colored (white, yellow; seldom red). The fruits are either dry, fine celled capsules or sour berries like little cucumbers. The former is the case with O. acetosella, which releases its seeds explosively, as does Impatiens or Touch-me-not.

Wood sorrels spread their over 350 species across the earth, mostly in the tropics and subtropics and none in cold zones; they are mostly herbs and seldom shrubs or trees. The main subfamily, Oxalis, has about 300 species, perennial plants with rhizome tubers or bulbs, palmate leaves with three to ten leaflets and white, yellowish and reddish flowers. They are joyful, green plants filled with sour juice, that like bushes, woods and other shady, moist places; O. natans (South Africa) even grow in the water. Over 30 species of Biophytum live in the tropics with leafy canopies of long and thin stemmed, pinnate leaves that close up like mimosas when they are touched. The long pinnate leaves of Averrhoa are also sensitive to touch; they are small trees whose inflorescence break directly out of the trunk, this is a tropical metamorphosis of the absence of shoots in wood sorrel, whose blossoms rise directly out of the rhizome. These blossoms on the trunk develop into finger long, sour fruits like little cucumbers that are a side dish on South American menus. The reader will have noticed that we spoke repeatedly about a particular substance in connection with the typical life of this interesting little family, namely, about oxalic acid. It is present in their juices in large amounts, together with potassium oxalate. That is how the acid got its name, but it is also present in substantial amounts in rhubarb, sorrel and many other plants, and in smaller amounts in all plants. Except that when they arise in the latter they are immediately exhaled again with the aid of a particular enzyme. Thus we have a universal and fundamental plant process here, which becomes manifest in the formation of oxalic acid, but which is more concerned with the activity that creates the acid than with the substance itself. All plants must generate oxalic acid, but only certain typical ones can accumulate them, and these include our wood sorrels.

This formation of acid occurs through an oxidation, an inner combustion of carbohydrate, which leads to carbon dioxide and water if it is carried to completion, but stops at the production of oxalic acid or other plant acids if it is only partial. Oxygen is the combustion agent. All biological processes are accompanied by breathing processes and a union with oxygen; life is a living flame. There is a lot of oxygen activity wherever strong life forces are developed. Young tissues breathe harder than old ones. Life and oxygen are connected with each other in a mysterious way. We have already indicated the direction in which one must look to get at the bottom of this mystery in this work, where we presented some interesting results of Rudolf Steiner's investigations. Oxygen is the mediating material and the portal for etheric, formative forces and for life in general. Life's formative forces and dead substances would exist side by side with no interaction between them, if oxygen would not be the great mediator. The supersensible realm of beings that is connected with the universal life forces that radiate in out of the universe press through the portal of oxygen and into the realm of earth forces and substances.

That is why congestions and stoppages in life processes are accompanied by congestions in oxygen activity.[21] This gives rise to incomplete inner combustion and to the formation of plant acids. All succulent plants accumulate such acids, especially at night when the sun's radiations and effects decrease and life quiets down. Of all the plant acids, oxalic acid is the most prominent product of such congestion.[22] The exhalation all the way down to carbon dioxide was stopped at the last possible step. Just compare its formula (COOH–COOH) with that of carbon dioxide (CO_2). This is a failure at the last minute.

---

[21] See the discussion in the section on Thick Leafed Plants – Grassulaceae
[22] The following chemical formulas of some plant acids are given for the reader's convenience: oxalic acid (COOH$_2$), tartaric acid COOH (CHOH$_2$), COOH, citric acid, aconitic acid, malic and COOH–COH, CHOH–COOH, succinic acid COOH (CH$_2$)$_2$ COOH, acetic acid CH$_3$COOH.

Thus we have a reduction in oxygen's efficiency and also a damming up of the normal course of the transformation of the uniformly blown up succulent shapes. However, wood sorrels are plants that are subjected to such biological congestions at first and then they overcome them and wrestle their way through to a normal plant shape.

Just as Oxalis acetosella must be placed between the two poles of etherically congested plants like sedums and astralized ones like peas with their butterfly flowers, so the formation of oxalic acid is a material event between etheric plant processes and astral, animal ones. Oxalic acid can easily be converted into formic acid (HCOOH). Animal organisms need this latter generation process but not the substance that arises from it, and so they excrete it. However, it is quite important in nature's whole household. In this respect ants are important organs of the earth being who by way of the ants create the amount of formic acid that is necessary for life on earth. In lectures on the nature of bees, Rudolf Steiner pointed to the really marvelous connection between the oxalic acid and formic acid processes in all earth life.

For the death side of all life requires that all things that have become corpses should be able to be transformed by the earth process in such a way that it can serve life again. Otherwise earth existence would eventually become a mummy and nature would have vainly "invented death in order to have a great deal of life."(Goethe)   Now ants are like organs for the whole of earth life that see to it that things that have died can become of use to life again. The earth recovers from its decomposition processes through their activity. This occurs in a very comprehensive way through the fact that they permeate the atmosphere with homeopathically diluted formic acid vapor that stimulates life in general and plant life in particular, and it doesn't just occur through the ponderable side of their activity. (People have rightly called ants the forests' health department.) Plants always develop in a healthier way if there are a lot of ants around, and they reactivate their oxalic acid process in connection with their biological development.

 But if the formic acid that is created means little to animals and is excreted in large amounts, why do they need the activity that generates formic acid? This question is connected with the secret of animal poisons in general. Modern spiritual investigation gives a surprising but deeply satisfying answer to this question, for it tells us that poisons are "collectors of the spirit". The poison process in the animal kingdom is connected with the intervention of animal spirituality in the bodies of certain animal genuses. In this Healing Plants we have often pointed to the connection of the poison process in the plant kingdom with the intervention of the plant's soul principle or astral sphere. Poisonous animals and plants are abnormal. If one looks around one notices that it is only the lower animals that get poisonous. There are no poisonous animals above reptiles any more. Thus poison is the way that spiritual formative forces have to go if they want to permeate an organism that stands at a stage of development that is too low for it to have made itself into a dwelling for these spiritual forces through an inner cosmos of perfect organs. "It is only because ants are constituted in such a way that they can generate formic acid, that everything they do seem to be so reasonable.

It is the ant colony as a whole that is so wise and not the individual ant." (R. Steiner, *Nine Lectures on Bees*).

* For the convenience of the reader, here are the chemical formulas of some plant acids:

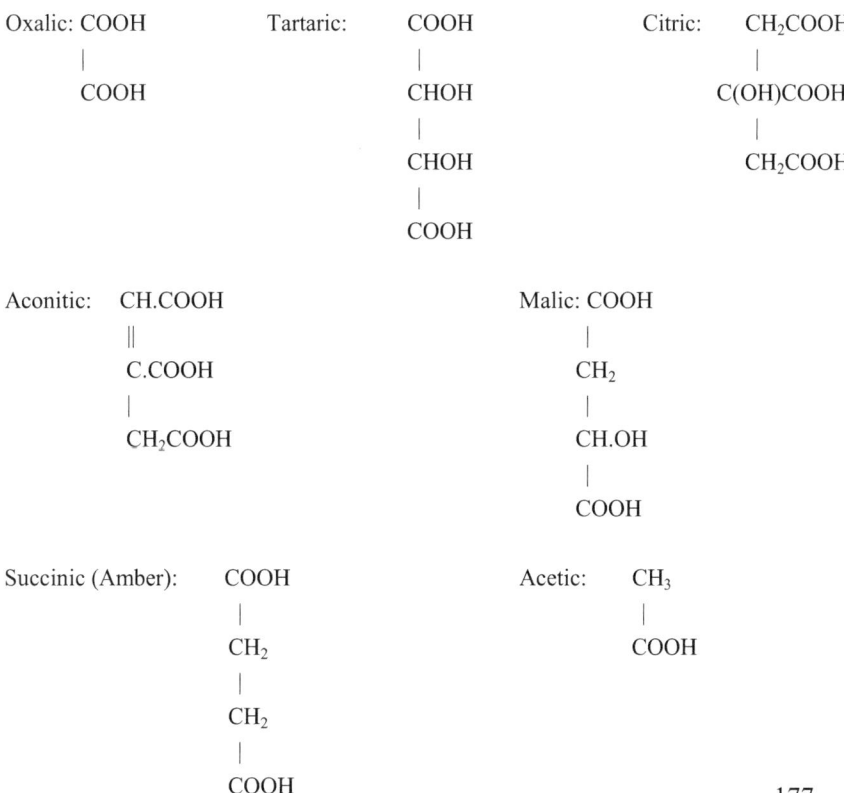

The human organization contains vegetative, vital processes and animal processes, or rather ones that are related to these two. Thereby it has processes that generate oxalic acid and other processes based on this that generate formic acid. The I or the spiritual part of man also lives in it. Thereby it contains a coordinated happening which occurs outside as a vegetative process that forms oxalic acid, as a process connected with ants that creates formic acid, as a pressing in of a spirited reality into events in nature from the universe, and as a wisdom interaction of these three realms of being. Living substance is constantly being made lifeless in human beings and in nature. The I organization needs this activity so that it can create the consciousness processes that are necessary for it. However, the lifeless things that are continuously formed for such purposes must be secreted by the astral body in a healthy way. The organism needs the production of formic acid to master this excretion in a healthy way. Gouty, rheumatic conditions arise if insufficient amounts are formed. The course is a certain stoppage of forces in the astral realm. A therapy without poison might be helpful here. However, an oxalic acid therapy would be appropriate if it is a weakness of the etheric that doesn't control the oxalic acid process properly and that results in a sluggish functioning of the liver, spleen and gall bladder, a tendency to form stones and the like.

Thus wood sorrel, that most impressive generator of oxalic acid, is a useful and fundamental remedy from the plant kingdom.

MALLOWS – MALVACEAE

The Formation of Mucilage and Fibers

The mallows are a medium sized family with over 900 species, most of which are natives of the tropics, although some of them also move into the temperate zones. They apparently want to unite with the earthy element with joyful, colorful gracefulness, and they protect themselves against hardening and lignification through the large amounts of mucilage they form. They leave most of the tree formation to the related Bombaceae, Sterculiaceae and Tiliaceae families, in which the soft wood and short, swollen, barrel shaped trunks tell one about a plastic, fluidic principle that is ever combating hardening lignification in them. However mallows generally remain herbs or shrubs. Their large, mostly bright colored flowers have something splendid but also mild about them. They shine but they don't glow, and they usually don't have much of an odor. They usually have a large number of stamens grown together into a tube in their five-petalled corollas, where the anthers protrude from the five main basic filaments through increasing divisions, and in some species they hang far out of the flowers. The leaves press into the flower formation and appear as a second calyx outside of the regular one. Their flowering process generally has a certain tendency to connect itself with the leaf region, and to glide down into it, for the flowers like to stand singly in the leaf axils. The leaves are also more or less attached to the stem, for they are either simple or palmately compound, there are no pinnately compound ones. The whole plant produces mucilage and the bark, phloem, stem and fruit of mallows develop particularly strong and excellent fibers. The family includes cotton and many other generators of spin-able fibers.

It is interesting that many good fiber plants produce mucilage. Good fibers are not lignified and therefore not brittle. This indicates that the production of mucilage must have something to do with the control of the lignifications process. The cellulose process is a metamorphosis of carbohydrate formation that is displaced towards the insoluble, solid side, and in the formation of wood it is connected with lignin, obtaining a mineral input from the roots. Plant mucilages are transformed cellulose. Water and some vitality are removed from carbohydrates in the formation of cellulose, for water is the bearer of vital formative forces. Life withdraws from wood and leaves a rigidified form of life behind. The opposite process or the tendency to hang on tight to the living watery element is present in mucilage formation. One can look upon the polarity between lignification and mucilage formation as a metamorphosis of the more primary polarity of starch and sugar formation, except that the first one has slipped one step lower. The primal process of assimilation that creates substances condenses carbon dioxide and water into starch under the influence of sunlight. At night this starch that is deposited in the grains of chlorophyll is taken hold of by the living fluidic system, combined with water, transformed into sugar, made soluble and handed over to the flowing sap region. The carbohydrate process swings back and forth between the formation of sugar and starch and the entry and exit of life forces (both of these go parallel with each other) it eventually swings out in fruit formation, as one gets sweet, juicy fruits in the one swing of the pendulum (prototype, grapes), and grains containing starch in the other swing (prototype, wheat). Bread and wine stand before us.

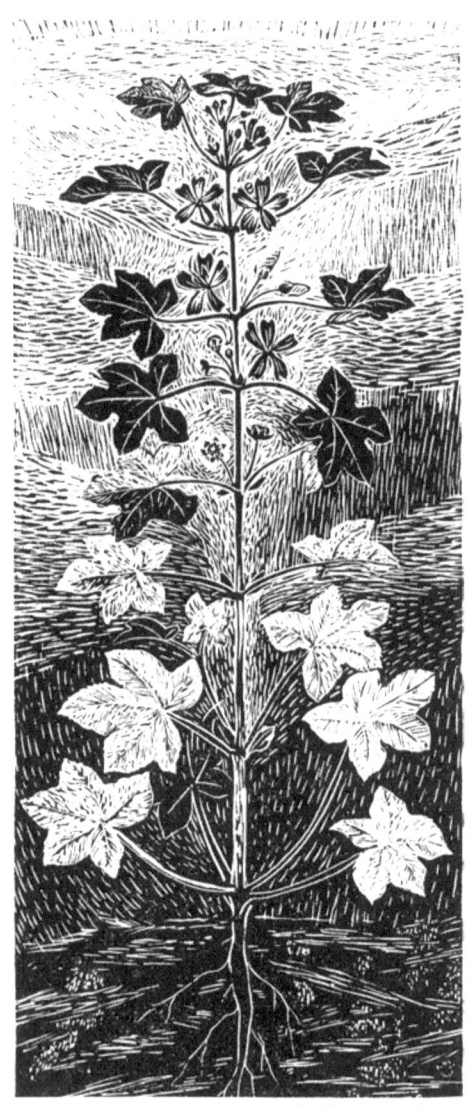

The pendulum doesn't swing back and forth in such a perfect way anymore one stage lower, for it gets into the region of hardening, material processes too much. Once something has fallen away from the realm of life forces and has become wood it generally has to stay wood. Only the very strongest forces of newly germinating life can reliquify the wood of a date kernel, for instance; or the etheric forces that are liberated by the wounding of a trunk can bring about a flow of gums. Therewith mucilage formations emerge as the opposite pole of wood formation where a plant protects itself against too much lignification through a concentration of its biological formative forces. Anyone who see the somewhat wooden, stiff magnificence of a crimson rambler or Papa Gontier with their large flowers will get the impression that they were made out of silk paper by a clever milliner and not out of live substances and he can tell himself that a delicate mucilage process permeates the plant from top to bottom and prevents the worst case, complete lignification.

Most mallow fruits are dry capsules, although some are permeated by mucilage processes, and in some species of hibiscus these processes are coupled with the formation of sugar and fruit acids to such an extent that the calyxes or whole fruits that become fleshy are eaten as soft vegetables in tropical lands or are preserved in vinegar. Our children like the mallow fruits that look like disks or Dutch cheeses.

The mucilage forming process which keeps the carbon process from getting stiff is also the one that makes hibiscus and other mallows into medicinal plants. The leaves, roots and blossoms are used internally and externally for the sake of their salutary mucilage that alleviates inflammations. Marshmallow root is an ingredient in many cough syrups, because of its decongesting and soothing effects upon the whole respiratory tract. The reader will see the extent to which plants that are involved with the carbon process a great deal have special connections with the lung organs, in the section on medicinal plants for organs that form protein and especially in the section about medicinal plants for the lungs.[23] Also see the discussion of mullein below.

The flowering process takes hold of the plant in such a gentle way in mallows that it does not permit the development of any poisonous species. There are also no parasitic plants or vines among them. In accordance with the threefolding key that the reader is already familiar with, the interaction of the flowering and leaf processes lead one to expect healing effects upon the human metabolic processes in the rhythmic system and upon the way that the astral body is active in this region. The inflammations and coughing reactions indicate that this member is cramped up; the remedy liberates it again.

One can also understand the soporific effect of mallow flowers from the effect of the flowering process that was mentioned (which arises through the influence of astral realms upon the plant's vegetative principle). In sleeplessness one has an inadequate ability to separate the astral body from the physical, etheric organization.

---

[23] See Typical Phenomenal Forms of Medicinal Plants for the Liver, Kidney, Lungs and Heart.

The above figure depicts Malva Sylvestris, subspecies mauritanica, a North African variety of our wild mallow or high mallow, whose flowers are used in the way just described.

*

SNAPDRAGONS – SCROPHULARIACEAE

The Type and a Few Medicinal Plants

Snapdragons look something like labiates outwardly, but they don't have the latters' strong warmth nature and they don't form essential oils. They are botanically close to the night shade family. Usteri put all three families in the Saturn subgroup of the highest, main group of flowering plants (the metachlamydeae, which belong to Venus as a group), namely in the tubiflorae.

♄ Saturn—Tubiflorae

♀ Venus—Boraginaoceae
♃ Jupiter—Labiatae
☿ Mercury—Verbenaceae
♂ Mars —Scrophularicae
☾ Moon—Hydrophyllaceae
☉ Sun—Solanaceae
♄ Saturn—Globulariaceae

Our type doesn't produce many shrubs and hardly any trees, but it creates quite a few semi-parasites that get part of their nourishment from other plant roots (e.g. yellow rattle, eyebright and cow–wheat). This indicates that they have a weak connection with the mineral, earth element. If the watery element predominates over the earthy one, our Scrophularias like it better and they then produce water side plants and aquatic ones in moors and swamps. They also do fine on well watered alpine meadows and wet pasture lands. Another thing they need is well lit air, and they look for it all the way up high in the mountains, where Alpine bartsia and mountain louseworts with reddish, violet and yellow tones unfold their flowering power in a cheerful and colorful way. Only the verbascums or mulleins grow on hot, dry, stony or sandy places and emphasize the vertical in their stems with a stiff and dry magnificence.

Close connections are made with the animal sphere that stands above plants if the roots and the relation to solid earth are somewhat weakly developed, and if the watery element is joyfully affirmed by juicy, possibly serrated, but not otherwise divided leaves so that the vegetative element is given its full rights. Animals are attracted to the many colorful manifold flowers even though they don't smell very much, and some of them have strange forms. These flowers choose the horizontal position and they thereby lose the all sided, radiant, basic form; they become symmetrical in two directions and thereby adopt a formative principle from animal bodies. In mulleins they are opened in a fairly flat manner (the mighty vertical stalk does not permit any other development), but in foxglove, brownwort and figwort they become deeply indented throats and in speedwells they are short tubular shells. The throats become bellies; in slipperworts one gets blown up, monstrous lower lips; the tendency to envelop the bubbles and to bring them into the flower's development becomes ever stronger until finally in hedge hyssops, antirrhinums, toad flaxes and cow wheats the throat closes entirely (only half way in eyebrights). The upper lip can also be pulled out into a monstrous trunk.

Thus the family strives towards the animal plant nature that is reminiscent of the animal plants on the old Moon, like several other families we've looked at, although in a particular way this time. Air as an incarnation element for the astral has a special connection with snapdragons, especially in their flowers. One doesn't see this striving towards aeriform things in the leaf region as much, except that species high up in the mountains grow delicate, pinnatified leaves.

For all of the intensity of the family's flowering process, the flowers are never pressed so strongly into the vegetative part that the latter is overpowered and paralyzed. The etheric sphere stops the on-storming astral element and masters and elaborates it. The flowers never grow at the end of a primary axis and take away the sprouting power of the main shoot, as happens so often in the nightshade family; one never gets a cramped, mutual proliferation of leaf, shoot and flower growth as one does in the latter. Such a strong family like the snapdragons does tend towards the formation of poisons but not to the formation of alkaloid poisons that contain nitrogen or to ones that tend to change one's consciousness. One will look for opiates and pleasurable poisons here in vain, although one does find saponines, and glycosidic poisons, and also bitter compounds. This means that the astral only influences the etheric and doesn't press down to the physical. Such poisons work into the nerve sense region less than the salty alkaloids do, but much more into the rhythmic region, which is involved with an interweaving of etheric and astral processes. The Scrophulariaceas are worked upon by what lies and weaves in between the fluidic and aeriform, and this also determines the kinds of conditions scrofula plants can address.

The fruits are usually capsules, seldom berries, with tiny, very light and sometimes winged fruits that blow around in the wind.

Scrofula plants mainly grow in the temperate rhythmic zones of the earth and even quite north and up in high mountains, but they stay away from deserts and the tropics. They have become important to men as medicinal plants, such as foxglove, eyebright, hedge hyssop, figwort, speedwell and woolly foxglove, and also as decorative plants that, however, look a little bizarre, deceptive and monstrous. An unbiased person quickly sees that all is not well with monkey flowers, snapdragons and slipperworts. The strong astralization makes the flowers a little frail and sometimes also a little short lived, which is partly compensated for by their large numbers. The colors are not very clear and pure, and the scents are poor. Nevertheless they are there in an intensive way and they force us to notice them. We will now describe some of the more important medicinal plants.

Digitalis purpurea – Foxglove

This plant's tiny seeds grow into a rosette of large, lanceolate, long stemmed leaves in the first year. The plant's growth is more in the strong root formation down into the earth, whereas the sprouting impulse towards the sun is held back. The counter thrust comes in the second year, a shoot is thrown straight up. The circle of leaves on the ground becomes a spiral on the rapidly rising stem, which becomes tightest as the leaves get shorter, until they creep into the mighty spikes as bracts and sepals. The flower buds that can be seen on these are spirally arranged and directed upwards. However, this basic arrangement changes when they open up. The flower that had previously been pointing in all directions now turns towards one side of the stem, and this is determined from outside, namely, by where the most light is coming from. They come down from their upright position to the horizontal and then even lower, and they point down and outward. The purplish red throats with delicate upper lips and massive lower lips open up; the upper sides flatten slightly and this makes them look like they've been inflated. It almost looks like too many

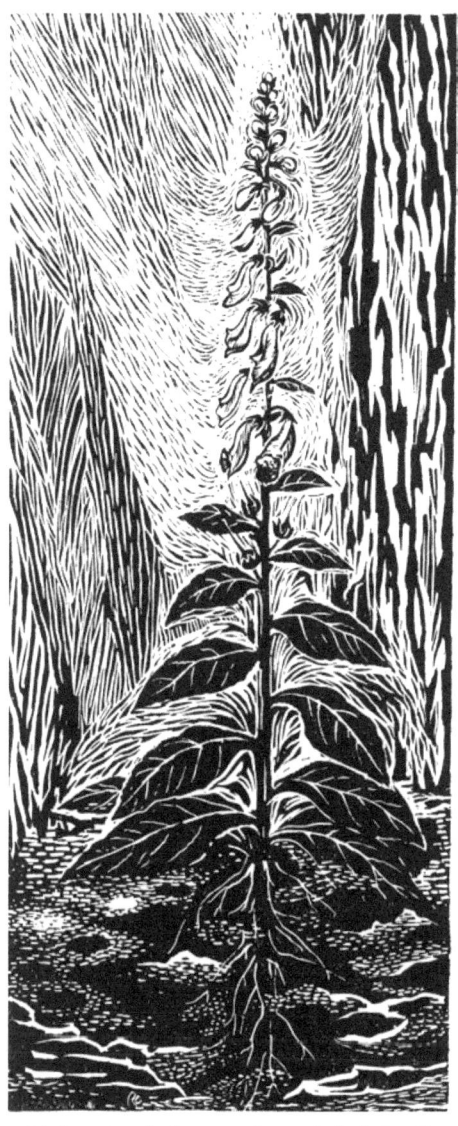

flowers are formed, the plant seems to be overpowered by the great weight of all the flowers.

The purplish red color is equally distributed inside the upper lips, and is in spots surrounded by a white border in the lower ones. The constricted base of this bell form contains the nectar that is in great demand by bees. The flower is short-lived and the inflated corolla falls off as if it had been cut by a knife. The heart shaped seed capsule and the calyx right themselves again. The storm of flowers that passed over the plant has cut into its vitality to such an extent that it usually dies at this point.

Thus after a foxglove turns towards the mineral earth that lies under it in a systolic contraction in the first year, it rises towards the animal realm above its plant nature in a diastolic exhalation of its forces in the second year, and it sinks into the horizontal plane into which animals have oriented their bodies and their main axis. The whole snapdragon family tends to have this orientation. Although the stem shoots up, borne by etheric levity forces, the astral realm that works in too strongly repels this etheric thrust, gravity takes hold of the flowers as they turn towards the light and the animalism opens up their throats in an excessive manner. Thus foxglove's life process is in a big battle between the polarities of light and gravity.

The digitalis process has its material expression in the formation of the so-called digitalis glycosides. Related substances that work strongly upon the heart can be found in Adonis, lily of the valley, strophanthus, oleander, squill and wall flower. These are all plants that place themselves and their life dynamics into the polarity of light and gravity with a strong tension between their etheric constitution or vitality principle and the astral realms that belong to them. (See what was said about these plants in Volume I, and see the section on medicinal plants for the heart in this volume.)

Although this group of substances occurs in the plant kingdom, it is very characteristic of it that it has its most manifold metamorphoses and greatest development in animal and human organisms. For instance one could mention toad poison, bufotoxin, here. Substances with similar structures are Vitamin D, cholesterol, bile acids and sex hormones. There is a sinister relative of these in the inorganic, coal tar realm that is carcinogenic, namely, benzopyrene. Of course coal also came from plants.

All of this points to processes that have to do with the interaction of the main plant and animal members, namely, of the etheric and astral ones. Foxglove poison and toad poison confront each other here. A toad is an amphibian that changes from a water animal with gills to an air animal with lungs, while it projects its limbs outwards and folds its air organ inwards. Practically blown up with air, the animal tries to fly up into the atmosphere, but it only manages to clumsily jump to get a fly or other insect. Amphibians are the first animals on the evolutionary ladder to find their voices. They can express their nature outwardly, albeit with a dull sound that is hung up in their metabolism and which corresponds to their awkward form of locomotion. Therewith amphibians acquire a capacity too soon, which the reptiles that stand above them are still lacking completely, and which only warm-blooded animals get. Amphibians are a lot like plants, with their skin opened up entirely to their environment, they are in tune with atmospheric life (which makes them into weather prophets); the inner and outer worlds stream into each other through their skin. Toads form a watery, glandular poison organ in this skin, and therewith set up a barrier to this intermingling of inner and outer. The group soul in lower animals that still works in from outside is in plants, it finds no proper organs for a real incarnation in the still imperfectly developed amphibian body, needs a toxic process in the physical and etheric bodies to latch on to. (This is why all poisonous animals are in the lower animal kingdom. A mammal that sucks up soul forces with its cosmos of perfected inner organs in a way that does justice to the world doesn't need such aids, which are only a makeshift situation.) One can see from toads that lower animals mainly need poisons for themselves, and not for doing harm to other organisms.

The pressing of the astral into the etheric body is a process that produces foxglove poison in the plant kingdom and toad poison in the animal kingdom. (That is why toads, unlike frogs, are unaffected by foxglove poison.)

One finds relatively high concentrations of so-called natural vitamin D (also called D3) and the related vitamin D2 that is formed in primitive animals in fishes' warmth organs or livers, in butter, milk and egg yolks, which points to a connection with organic warmth processes. They work strongly in the metabolism of calcium and phosphorus and on the structure of bones; if too much of this is present, the calcium process is displaced from the bones into vessel walls and inner organs, and it would like to sclerotize the blood man, as it were. In healthy bone formation the most spiritual part of man, his I, forms the physical and almost mineral bones, makes a copy of itself in them, and therewith places itself entirely into the material, earthly region and into the realm of the dead, although it is a spiritual being. To this end it dampens living warmth processes, brings organic "cold" into the region in which the bones are supposed to form, unites itself with mineral lawfulnesses and their formative powers and almost at the edge of the minerally dead kingdom, it forms that marvelous skeleton that is a dead image of the I and that retains the "trace wrought by God" (Goethe) for a long time after death. Thus Vitamin D is the instrument for a process that incarnates or presses the spirit into the physical. (There lies the danger in using this remedy for rickets on all babies, as our overzealous health personnel would like to do. One should let the incarnating I carry out this delicate process and form the instruments for this by itself as much as possible, and at most help it out where it proves to be too weak, but one shouldn't brutally prevent its effort to form its own instruments. Otherwise the incarnating human being is deprived of its childhood, is cut off from its heavenly, spiritual origin too soon and is made too earthy.)

The bile acids that are generated by the warmth organ, the liver, and excreted into the intestine, open up fats and cholesterol in food for digestion. (Only plant sterols remain indigestible.) Thereby they are split up in the small intestine (into cholic acid and glycine or taurine) and then absorbed by the body together with the digested fats. They then wind up in the liver and are recombined with glycine or taurine and are handed over to the bile. Thus the fluid organism exhales bile acids in order to take hold of the fats that bear warmth in the intestine, and it inhales them and the transformed fats again. The latter bring nothing of the foreign organization from which they came into the human organization except for the ability to generate warmth.[24] Plants created them through cosmic warmth processes and by developing a lot of hydrogen forces, especially in their seeds, and they separated these from earthly, gravity processes and exposed the creative chaos in seed protein to the formative cosmic regions and to nothing else. The origins of all material things that descended out of the spiritual world into matter are in warmth. Thus in a way fats are warmth that has become material (see the introductory sections in Volume I). They isolate physical forces from the world of gravity and they let in the world of levity, etheric forces and especially warmth ether. The I and astral body work into the fats in foods through bile acids in order to place them in the service of the warmth organization, that shapes the whole body in an interplay of warming and cooling processes between dissolution and hardening.

Cholesterol is a waxy substance that can crystallize into rhombic plates; it is insoluble in water and soluble in fats. It is found in the blood, brain, bile and egg yolks. As an ester of fatty acids it is found in wax, blood, lymph, brain, adrenal glands, corpus luteum, epidermis, skin fat (and woolfat), in the vermix on new born infants, in all horny substances, hair, feathers, hoofs, where the sulfur process that pushes into the silica sphere produces horn (Rudolf Steiner said that the hydrogen process is the most important in horn). Cholesterol is practically pure hydrogen and carbon, with only one part oxygen, according to the empirical formula, $C_{22}H_{46}O$.

In cholesterol the fat, wax, warmth and hydrogen process takes in cold and form impulses from the senses and nerve spheres. That is why

---

[24] See Ita Wegman, Rudolf Steiner, *Fundamentals of Therapy*

one gets deposits and stonelike formations of cholesterol in deposition and hardening diseases (in the vascular walls in sclerosis and in the gall bladder in gall stones).

One finds the so-called sexual hormones (androsterone, testosterone, follicle hormone and corpus lutetium hormone) connected with processes that have to do with the function of sexual organs and their rhythms. During fertilization the egg cell's protein is made chaotic and inwardly fractured, raised out of earthly processes and exposed to the cosmos. The etheric forces that have been specialized by the spiritual members of the human being that is descending out of the spiritual world into the physical, earthly world radiate in from the cosmic periphery. They mediate body forming impulses to this chaotic, germinal protein, which is therefore capable of being formed and determined in an almost limitless way. We have another hydrogen process at work here, through which matter withdraws from terrestrial forces and opens itself to the cosmos. Rudolf Steiner also showed to what extent a woman's uterus is a metamorphosed heart whose solar rhythms are adapted to the lunar, sexual sphere, and is therefore transformed accordingly.

*

This is how one can begin to understand the connections between things like cardio-glycosides, toad poison, bile acids, cholesterol, sexual hormones and vitamin D_3. Their common denominator becomes perceptible. The substance that withdraws from the earthly realm of forces in the hydrogen process is opened to the realm of cosmic formative forces, and the higher spheres or members (depending on whether plants, animals or humans are involved) are practically forced to intervene or to incarnate. This gives such substances a strong effect that can easily get too strong and that can end in one's being too deep into one's body and in a fettering and hardening in this or that direction.

One will now be better able to understand the way that foxglove poison affects the heart. It lets the astral body intervene more intensively into the fluidic organism and especially into blood circulation in the veins and it makes the latter less heavy and gives it a good tone. Thereby dieresis is enhanced. Edemas are flushed out, the blood pressure rises and the heart's systolic action is strengthened. One sees a strengthening of that contracting force which the blood exerts on the heart through its calcium content (whereas potassium promotes the opposite, diastolic process). Therewith we come back to the calcium process that we noticed when we were looking at vitamin D and the action of cholesterol, except that now it is now in the blood. Too much digitalis poison contracts the heart and stops it.

Rudolf Steiner never recommended the use of foxglove as a heart remedy, he mentioned primula, onopordon, carduus benedictus, paeonia officinalis and others for this purpose instead. (See the description of these in this book.)

Euphrasia officinalis [25] - *Eyebright*

This humble little plant fits itself into the community of plants on our meadows in its own way. The lush life on meadows owes its basic tone to grasses. As the latter send up one node after another they develop a strong vitality with respect to the earth. They suck up the watery element strongly into their sprouting freshness and they drive their narrow long leaf spears up into a sea of light, like rays, in anticipation of the stems that, bear the spike of flowers that are wind fertilized and entirely adapted to the airy element. Grass plants rise powerfully in the realm of light and air, but they develop little color or scent. Grasses' high content of silica and carotene is connected with their love of light.

Eyebright selects this strong life process in the earth region as the foundation for its roots, and it roots semi–parasitically upon the grass roots thereby dampens the grasses' life and directs it into its own growth processes that drive it up to blossom and fruit in one year. This decreases grass growth, which is why one used to scold eyebright for being a hay rogue and a milk thief. Its small shoot with paired, ovate, slightly serrated leaves rapidly passes over into a fairly large number of flowers. The flowers that appear one after another and that look out horizontally sit in the axils of the leaves around the stem; a rhythmic leaf system and flowering process press into each other. The inflorescence stretches up slowly and develops one pair of flowers after another from the end of May until October. It keeps on growing and blooming. Thus the flowering process places itself in the midst of growth development. The flower arches its violet upper lip and protrudes its white lower lip that is

---

[25] Collective name for E. Stricta and E. Rostkowiana

decorated with dark streaks and a bright yellow spot in the throat; it is like a moderated, toned down inflammation. It displays color and counter color, just as our eye when it looks at a yellow color, immediately generates a violet in itself as a complementary and balancing color, in order to equilibrate and free itself with respect to the compulsion of sensory stimuli. When the eye sees both color and complementary color in the outer world, it feels sympathetically moved by something that is harmonious, and this may be why the sight of this plant is so appealing.

An eye sits in the upper organization like a semi parasite that is rooted there (and that is why it can be removed in severe diseases); Rudolf Steiner pointed to a strange similarity between eye formation and the organic processes that occur in combustion. According to Goethe's explanations in his *Color Theory*, light once brought out the organ that is appropriate for it "from indifferent organs", and Steiner said that it took hold of the organism with incendiary force, which responded with processes that are somewhat similar to those in combustion. The organism created its eyes in a creative synthesis of action and reaction, and one can clearly see that they were shaped from two sides, from outside (lens, iris, vitreous humor) and from inside (retina, veins, nerves). An eye is like a healed inflammation that is withdrawn from subjective feelings (it is beyond pleasure and pain). It senses light and colors in an objective way, and it has become factual in its sensations. When it gets inflamed from colds it falls back into its old condition; too many metabolic processes press towards it, the astral body mediates too few objective light and form forces, and it wallows in the subjective pain sphere. Euphrasia dampens the etheric forces of its environment, upon which it lives parasitically, and it discloses its snapdragon nature through its flowers. That is, how it is permeated by astral forces, and it can relieve the organism from the abnormal activity of its members, that becomes manifest in inflammations from colds, in which an excess of springing metabolic activity is opposed by the little formative power. Thus Euphrasia works upon the stomach's mucous inflammations, regulates the intervention of the astral body in this region, and also combats eczemas and other skin diseases, in which an irregular metabolism presses too strongly into the skin's sensory sphere. However, since the whole Euphrasia process attaches itself parasitically to the grasses' root region, this gives a special connection with the upper organization, and through the strong silica process connects one another to the organs that mediate light. Thus one can understand its good effect upon inflammations and colds in the sheaths surrounding the eyes, in inflammations of the connective tissue with many tears, conjunctivitis, blepharitis and iritis.

Among the material impressions of life processes that chemists have found in eyebright are tannins (that are connected with an attraction of the astral sphere), etheric oils, aromatic resins (copies of gentle warmth processes in this summer plant) and aucubine, a special glycoside that also occurs in a few other snapdragons attracted to light and meadows. This is a material expression of an abnormally strong intervention of the astral sphere into the middle rhythmic region in snapdragons, with a weakening of the root sphere that connects them with the earth. This glycosidic poison generates a corresponding headache, dizziness, bleeding in the brain and inflammations in the gastro-intestinal tract; metabolic processes (that are especially stimulated by the blood region) overpower the nerve-sense region that is ascribed to the root region.

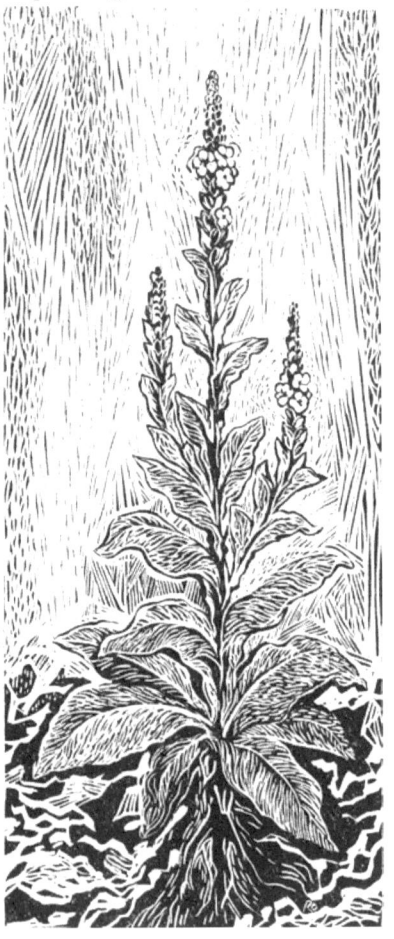

Verbascum Thapsiforme – Mullein

There are over 200 species in the mullein genus that are mostly native to the sunny, hot, dry, eastern Mediterranean region, including our stately great mullein. The latter loves stony, dry, warm, growing places, rocky, southern exposures on hills, river gravel and similar soils. The biennial plant develops a rosette of undivided, woolly, long and wide leaves with petioles; it bores down deep into the ground with its mighty main root. At this stage one could get a remedy from its root that would work upon one's head. What was held on the ground shoots stormily into the vertical in the second year and rises so energetically that the leaf formation is swept along like wings up the stalk, especially if the latter gets very tall, except for the ends of the leaves until it winds down as bracts at about the height of a man. This flower candle is the imposing, regal, main organ that develops large numbers of large, bright yellow flowers with orange veins in the hot days of July and August. They look out towards the sides, and are therefore flat and asymmetrical, so that the three lower petals are the largest, and they are pasted on a thick, gray felt, central rod, a sunny yellow and festively shining sacrificial candle on a stony altar in honor of a summer's day. Since this rhythmic flower stem that swallows up leaves is the main organ, one would expect it to have metabolic effects in the rhythmic system.

The dry plant's flowers are not exactly dripping with nectar, but it drives sugars into its petals and especially into the stamens where insects like to feed; it avoids woody rigidification by developing a lot of mucilage which permeates the whole plant right into the flower petals. The carbohydrate process is protected from excessive lignification and it points to the lungs as the healing region, as we will explain later. [26]Its dried, slimy, sweet flowers are an important component of chest teas. Metabolic processes that work too strongly into the lungs and the rest of the rhythmic system in inflammations due to colds are counteracted by the dynamics of the mullein process which facilitates the elimination of mucus. The plant's saponin content also helps here as explained elsewhere in this book.

Veronica officinalis – Speedwell

The snapdragon family attains its finest forms in the over 200 species of speedwell that live in temperate and cool climates. New Zealand in particular has a lot of strange species such as bushes with evergreen leaves. The parasitic element is overcome and the various forms of speedwell live in the woods, meadows, fields, pastures and banks of the cooler parts of the temperate zone. Their delicate, ephemeral, mostly blue flowers in large numbers are only slightly asymmetrical, flat disks. The

---

[26] See the chapter on the typical properties of plants that heal the liver, kidneys, lungs and heart.

impulse to form throats, snouts and deep tubes that are dark yellow, insistent orange or striped red and purple has disappeared. The shoots creep along the ground with many branches. The flowers in the leaf axils are taken into this onflowing growth. Or else short racemes rise up from the axils. In the best kinds the whole shoot stands up, the leaves change into small bracts and the blue flower spikes stand out in a distinctive way. That is what a spiked, long leafed speedwell looks like.

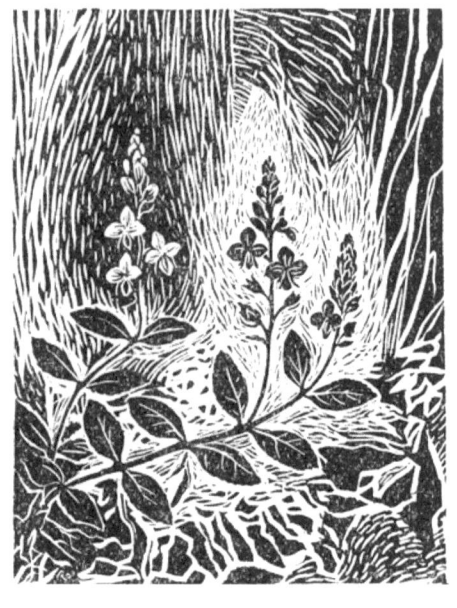

The genuine speedwell or forest variety didn't get quite as perfect. The shoot creeps along out of the perennial rootstock for quite a distance, sending out little roots out of the nodes. The opposite, somewhat thick little leaves are oval and slightly serrated. As one gets closer to the flowers, side shoots lift up out of the leaf axils, there is still one or two pairs of leaves, and then it goes into the stiff, upright cluster of flowers with their four petaled, flat, pale violet, ephemeral blossoms that bloom from June to August. The triangular, little seed capsules contain many, tiny seeds. We find our plant at the edges of woods and woodpaths. It likes the dimmed light around tall trunks in woods.

In Veronica officinalis the vegetative leaf and stem element plays with the flowering principle that eventually takes hold of it strongly and devitalizes it. It only puts out tiny sepals and only permits each flower to live a short time. But it is quickly replaced by a new one. Thus the etheric nature of the plant attracts snapdragons' strong astral impulse that takes hold of the plant and devitalizes it and permeates it with poison. However the etheric part evens this out so that it is only a slight permeation with poison that produces glycosides but no alkaloids. Such a dynamics results in the formation of bitter substances. These substances make the etheric body inclined to unite with the astral sphere, as we mentioned in Volume

I for gentians. The basic condition for a healthy breathing process is a proper, rhythmic uniting and separating of the astral body and etheric body. According to Rudolf Steiner, if the astral body is unable to let go properly in exhalation, asthmatic symptoms result. He said that one can combat this by the alternate administration of tannins and Veronica bitters. These take hold at the other end, that is, they make the astral body inclined to unite itself with the etheric body, as we also pointed out in numerous places in Volumes I and II. [27]However, asthmatics do not have this healthy connection; their organisms don't have the necessary "opposite"; the right connection between the etheric organization and the astral organization is interrupted, "for this is what a lack of appetite means." (Rudolf Steiner, lecture of January 2, 1924, GA 314) An asthmatic has no appetite in his whole organism. "He has no desire to take foodstuffs into those parts that pass over into the entire circulation."

We tried to show that we have a special astralization of the rhythmic system in snapdragons and a stunting of their connections with the earth. This is overcome in speedwell species towards both the flower and the root sides. Anyone who has looked at the greedily sucked up, inflated air formation of a slipper flower with a certain uneasiness, feels better when he sees the liberated openness of a speedwell flower. The latter can become an image for the cured pathological interactions of etheric and astral impulses that are present in most Scrophulariaceae.

Gratiola officinalis – Hedge Hyssop

Here the archetype of the snapdragons dives down into the damp element, to the extent that it is well illuminated. Hedge hyssop's fleshy, 1/4 inch thick rhizome penetrates swampy meadows, turf moors and wet soils along rivers and seas. The shoot goes up vertically to about knee height. The leaves are opposite, sheathing, lanceolate and grass-like. The tubular, two lipped, long peduncled flowers grow out horizontally from the leaf axils, and they look cheerful with their red stripes on a white background; five delicate, pointed sepals flutter around their bases. Node follows node in rhythmic fashion, the flowering and leaf elements intermingle and flow along the stem, determined by the fluidic element in the soil although they do permit light and air to be fully active.

---

[27] See the index under astral.

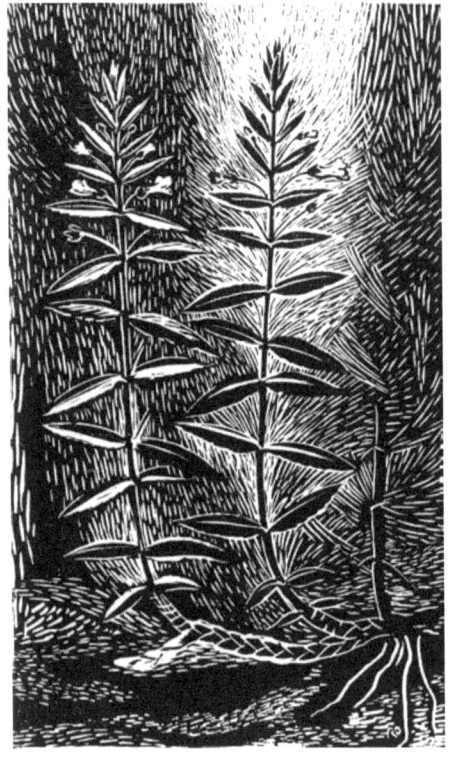
The pointed little seed capsules contain tiny seeds. The flowers open in the summer months.

After observed sympathetically the rhythmic stem formation and the leaves that change very little from top to bottom, and seeing how the flowers fit themselves into this pattern, one is surprised that the flowers strive away from the stem with long peduncles. A second formative motif is expressed in them. If one imagines the stem with leaves but no flowers, and then imagines the reverse with only pairs of flowers at each of the upper nodes, one will develop an organ for the perception of the transformative power that leads from one formative motif to the other.

In accordance with its "signature", the plant works strongly into the rhythm of the metabolism, since its shoot has this mixture of rhythmic, etheric leaf processes on an astrally conditioned flowering process. It has a good effect on colds in the intestine, painful diarrhea and colics, and the astral body is stimulated into gaining a better control over a digestive system that has become atonic. Gratiola is also used for skin eruptions, because they are an expression of an irregular metabolism that works into the region of the nerve sense system. Our plant is also helpful in cases with psychological symptoms that result from congestions of man's higher members in his liver and other metabolic organs. The oral intake of a few drops of its mother tincture enhances the eye's ability to perceive green, whereas if the dose is increased they can no longer perceive it, which is a strange phenomenon. The activities of light and darkness are balanced in green, the equilibrated color. This creative balance of color disappears for someone who has been poisoned by Gratiola; the green looks like a passive gray to him, the activities of light and darkness proceed side by side uncreatively and they don't interact in a forceful way.

The specific life processes of such a plant have their material imprints, of course; chemists find the glycoside gratioline, small amounts of gratiotoxine that has a similar effect to that of digitalis, and very bitter substances. The effects of gratioline are cruder than the more encompassing effect of the whole plant.

Scrophularia nodosa – Figwort

Here we are pointed to damp and dark places like bushes, ditches in the woods, and shady river banks. A shoot and its leaves that looks like a nettle rises 2–3 feet from a short, powerful root stock that has swollen into an ovate nodule at the node and up above it passes over into a panicle of terminal flowers. The latter separates itself resolutely from the nettle–like leaves and distances itself from the pairs of leaves that have towered up on one node after another. This stripping off of something lower leads upwards but not into the light; the flowers with their swollen corolla tubes and dismal, dark brown and olive green throats that look gloomy tell us something about the forces of darkness that are working into them. The crushed herb has a damp, burnt smell. Its ovate capsules contain many tiny seeds. Figwort blooms in the summer, like most other snapdragons.

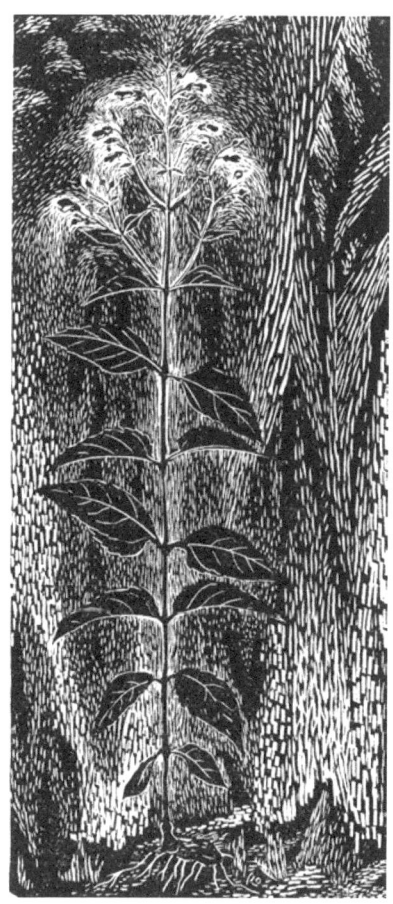

The plant contains saponins, flavones and some digitalis glycosides. Our medicinal plant's name points to its healing effect upon scrofulous, tuberculous skin and glandular diseases in children. The plant has also been used in the treatment of ulcers, eczemas in the head region and goiter, like many other plants that have congested vitality in their root regions, as one can see from the nodular swellings (as in autumn crocus, cyclamen and crocus). The mastery of bubbling dampness, the battle with insufficient light, the successful astralization and the transformation of the leaf process into the inflorescence that is all by itself on the top give the healing connection with scrofulous processes, in which a bloated organism that isn't shaped enough etherically, does not adequately permeate itself with light and astrality.

BINDWEEDS – CONVOLVULACEAE

One gets a good idea about the bindweed type if one follows the growth of field bindweed or of hedge bindweed, since both of these plants express it in a characteristic way. The great vitality in their much divided root stocks that suck out the earth realm, and the roots that grow exuberantly through the ground, gather together into nests and creep along in long strings, ready to produce a whole plant out of each little piece; this makes morning glory plants into bad weeds. Once the rising shoots break through the surface of the ground they manage to work their way upwards by winding around other plants, since bindweeds can't do this by themselves. Short stemmed, unserrated and undivided sagittate leaves that often point upwards climb to this serpentine line; beautiful, large, pale colored, often fragrant, funnel form flowers with long peduncles; the life of the leaves presses up into the flower region and can even envelope the fruit by growing on in the calyx. Each flower is short lived and withers fast, but is replaced by another one just as quickly. Thus the strong vitality of the root region flows through the extensively divided shoot and up in to the flower region. However, there is a threshold there as the astral sphere reveals itself, mightily, and demands the sacrifice of the lower in order to produce the higher, beautiful, showy flowers. Mercury, active in many ways in the upwardly winding snake staff opens up Venus' life petals in the flower chalices.

The type produces more than 1100 species and spreads them over the earth, although most of them live in the tropics. Many are weeds and many are decorative plants, due to the beauty of convolvulaceae plants in general. The lower element that is rampant in the upper region produces sweet, fleshy fruit stems in some species and berries in others, but mostly dry capsules. The root stems of goat foot bindweed burrow through the sand dunes of tropical islands for 30–40 meters. Others wind their way up trees for several meters, and all have beautiful, colorful and fragrant flowers, and all are graceful. Batatas, the sweet potato of the tropics, has brought its fruit forces down into the root region; side roots swell up into fist sized tubers that contain a lot of starch.

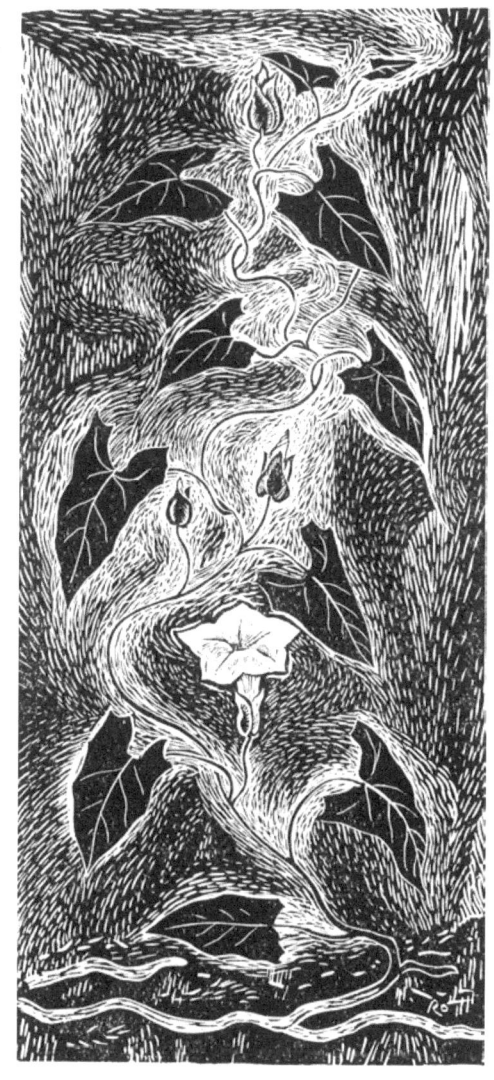

The 100 species of cuscuta that include the clover and nettle dodders at our latitudes have a different one–sided development of the type. All of its forces are concentrated in the stem region, just as they are localized in the root region in sweet potatoes and goat foot bindweeds. The winding stem sends suckers into the supporting, upright host to draw out its transformed earth juices, and its own roots and leaves die. The small, flesh red thickish flowers bunch up into little clusters, and the plant mainly becomes a parasitic bunch of flowers that gets its roots, stems and leaves from the other "normal" plant.

The convolvulaceae tell us something about their nature through the substances they form, and these include strongly working resins called "scammony," which are obtained by incisions into the root stalk of the oriental purging bindweed, and also from dodders and our local bindweeds. Jalap roots and resins from the Mexican, cathartic, bindweed Ipomoea purga, the scammony resin just mentioned, and the resinous glycoside that is present in field bindweed and hedge bindweed (known as scammonium germanicum) are all used as purgatives. One can expect effects upon the metabolic rhythms because of the interaction of the rhythmic stem process and the flower process. The "sulfuric" flowering processes that thrust down into the stem and roots and rigidify there as resins can accelerate peristalsis and make the contents of the intestines more aqueous by excreting fluids from the body's interior into them. The resorption process is opposed by a secretion process, and something that tends to dry out in the metabolism becomes vitalized; on the other hand, the subconscious perception of the products of digestion, that should be excreted, is enhanced by the resins that represent a sulfuric element that has become too physical and completely undigestible.

Anyone who looks at the spirally winding shoot that puts out an almost endless number of nodes and leaves will see its mercurial nature. Bindweed resins have a good effect on the same region that mercury compounds do, namely, where the quicksilver, Mercury process is active in the convoluted intestinal organ at the points where the liquefied chyme goes into the body's interior. Sulfuric substances in the Mercury region have a salutary effect.

THE OLIVE FAMILY – OLEACEAE

The Process that Forms Oils in the Plant Kingdom

The members of the olive family are so different and manifold that at first the type seems to stay concealed behind the large number of outer forms. Just try to find the common denominator for olive trees, ashes, lilac, privet, forsythia and jasmine. One has to understand mighty tree formations, a going up into blossoms and scents, and the peaceful collected state of a delightful oil giver on the basis of one spiritual principle, and it is not easy to find.

*

The tall, stately and well illumined ash with its delicately shaped pinnate leaves, white, elastic wood and winged seeds swinging in the wind, shows us earthly substances that have let themselves be taken hold of and lifted up by the transformative forces of cosmic light regions. The ash is just as much of a light and sun tree as the oak is a Mars and earth tree. An old weather rule said that one should observe which of the two – ash or oak – put out shoots first in the spring. A year that is greeted by greening ash twigs will become a hot and dry sun year, whereas a year that is welcomed by green oak parts first will be a very wet one. Our ancestors saw an ancient condition of the earth shining through ashes when the heavenly bodies and the sun and earth were still united; they spoke of the World Ash, Yggdrasil that still contained all creatures in its large living organism. The first pair of still quite plantlike humans, Ask and Embla, were born from this vital cosmos that was permeated by the sun's force, where Ask, the old word for ash, was the Adam in this myth.

The second pair of columns under the large cupola of the first Goetheanum which Rudolf Steiner built, were made of ash. They represented the story of evolution that he called the "old Sun evolution" in his books and lectures.

The ash genus gives an excellent wood, and also waxy and honey-like substances. Among its 40 some species is the Manna ash that leaks out sweet manna (mannitol, a sugar alcohol with six hydroxyl groups) from wounds that are made by manniferous cicadas or by man; this is a mild purgative (The wax louse feds on the Chinese ash.) using "Chinese wax" as a protective sheath for its offspring.

At a time when wise men knew how to express deep insights in fairy tale pictures, a feeling for the light and sunny character of ashes made them ascribe an ability to ash to drive away snakes and to protect one from lightning to ashes. The faith that ashes give healing forces also comes from such an experience. People kept some ash wood on their clothes or around their necks so that wounds would heal faster. They tried to combat intermittent fevers with the bark, and gout and rheumatism with its leaves.

Syringa, the lilac shrubs and small tree genus with over 30 species from Japan to eastern Europe, is a hard wood and a photophilic plant, but it tries to develop showy flowers on every branch and twig. It does not dissolve its inflorescence into the air and wind like the ashes that renounce color and scent and flashy corollas. However, its magnificence is a little bit stiff, for it participates in its vigorous inflammation of flowers with a somewhat melancholic joyfulness. It is a joyful outburst that is dampened by a quiet sadness, although it is a fragrant inflammation that is very intense. The corollas have long tubes and insects are attracted by a fair amount of nectar that flows at their bottoms. On the other hand, in ashes, brownish, dried out capsules remain after their flowers have burned out, which is a withered contrast to their fresh, green, tree–crowns.

Rudolf Steiner once recommended the use of lilac blossoms (or elderberry flowers) for upper respiratory tract infections. As in the case of ashes, syringa bark and leaves were once used as antipyretics.

Jasmine is the largest genus in the family with over 200 species. They get into a sweet, fragrant flowering process to an even greater extent than lilacs do. They are mostly shrubs in the warm zones of all continents, and they are used in perfumes, as a spice in certain teas, for making flower necklaces or leis, and as a votive offering, depending on the tribe and cultural region concerned. They are only mentioned here in order to elucidate a characteristic feature of the Oleaceae family. These fragrant bushes develop berries with oily seeds.

One has to approach the olive tree with reverence, for it is not only a giver of food and one of the oldest, cultivated plants, it is also an aid in healing, a giver of substances for cultic rituals, for the consecration of kings and priests, and for the last annointment. It is the priestly patriarch among trees; the ceremoniousness and the great peacefulness of a sacred place in nature lives in the luminous shade of an olive tree grove that is now gently woven through by silver and now by flashes of bright gold. The peoples of the eastern Mediterranean, where it originally came from, felt that it was a gift straight from the gods, especially the Greeks, who thanked Athena for giving them their first oil tree, and it would have been an unthinkable crime to cut olive trees down.

Olive trees take hold of the solid, hard earth with tremendous vitality and force; they especially like rocky, sunny hills and mountain sides. They are covered with dormant eyes on their roots and trunks from which they can put out shoots and rejuvenate themselves; branches that touch the ground can also take root. Even if an ancient trunk splits apart like an old willow stump, and even if it looks more like a crumbled rock or a ruin then a plant formation, new shoots will come out of it every spring. Olive trees make it particularly clear that a tree is really protruding earth, which in this case is earth that is almost as hard as a rock. However this part of the earth is particularly open to the cosmos' light and warmth nature.

Olive trees create a biosphere that is continually played through by light and warmth, by the way their branches and crowns are formed and through the willowy, narrow, lanceolate, evergreen leaves that are gray green above and shiny silver below. It is not just through the fact that for their home they have chosen a lot of sunshine and "bright" warmth and the climatic zone that is harmonized by the Mediterranean Sea. They stay away from shady, damp and dark areas, showing themselves even in the silvery, greenish gray color of their trunks.

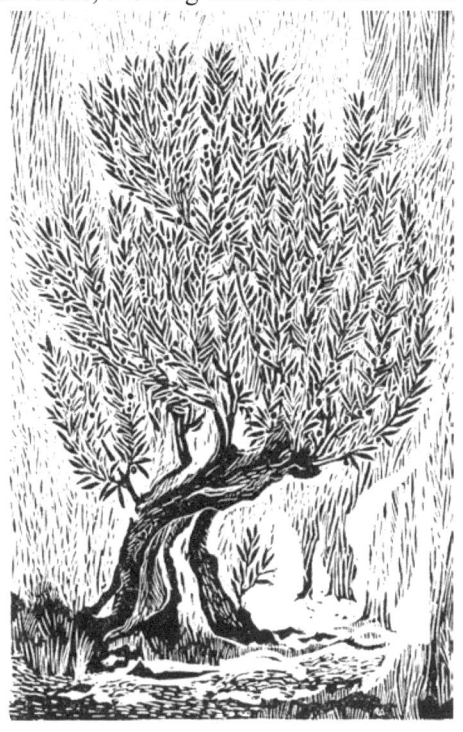

Their privet-like, small, delicate, yellowish white flowers break out of the leaf axils in short racemes in April and May, which is almost like summer in the Mediterranean. They have a delicate, modest fragrance. Like sloes, their fruits ripen slowly; the tree sends its whole vitality into their formation and ripening, for it grows very little during this time. It stops growing and sprouting almost entirely during harvest time, which lasts from late fall until the end of winter. What ashes use for tall growth, and jasmines use to direct their intoxicating fragrance outwards, is held fast inside olive trees and used in a different direction. That is why olive trees can get so ancient. It is possible that some of the trees in the Garden of Gethsemane under which Jesus Christ walked and stayed during the hours that began His Passion are still standing today.

The process of oil formation occurs more perfectly in olive trees than in most other plants. Oil formation is a basic process in the plant kingdom that definitely belongs to plant existence, although it occurs somewhat differently in each species, and therefore is something universal and specific at the same time. Poppy oil is different from hazelnut oil or sesame oil. Linseed oil, gourd oil, sunflower oil, peanut oil, palm kernel oil and coconut oil each have a particular quality.

Oil is the substance with which a plant closes off its life cycle during the ripening of its seeds, it therewith retreats again from the sensory world into the world of being, just as water is the substance with which the plant being must unite itself in order to leave the supersensible realm of beings and enter and appear in the sense world. All plants that form seeds contain oil in their germs, and quite a bit of wheat germ oil and corn–germ oil is being consumed today. Many plants go beyond the germ and fill the whole seed with oil, as in almonds and in cherry and peach pits. However, a few go all the way and make the whole fruit oily, not just the germ and seeds such as sea buckthorn, avocado, oil palms, and the queen of all fruit trees that produce oil, namely, our olive tree.

A few deciduous trees in our region with soft woods like birches and lindens undergo a peculiar metamorphosis of this fat production in the seed and fruit region. When they have closed off their life cycle in the late fall, produced and discarded their flowers, fruit and leaves and withdrawn into bud formation, and have gone to sleep for the winter, they fill their wood with a delicate fat formation, which disappears again when things begin to sprout in the spring, just as the oil in seeds is transformed to something else when they germinate. Hard woods and shrubs that have been hardened under the influence of earthly forces can form no fats.

Gentians and other perennials form fatty oils in their roots in the late fall. Thus generally speaking, the beginning of growth stands under the sign of water and the end of growth stands under the sign of oil.

Therewith one has grasped the secret of oil formation. One gets additional insight if one follows the path of the warmth effect in the plants' life. Warmth activity always permeates the various phases of plant development from outside because plants don't have man's inner warmth organization. However, plant life is taken hold of by cosmic warmth forces in a stepwise manner. The germination process requires a certain warmth that must have been conveyed to soil and water, and this also stimulates and accelerates the life processes indirectly. If a pumpkin or other plant species sucks in excess warmth forces at the stage when the watery element predominates, its shape swells up and its growth becomes bloated and monstrous. Sharp, fiery juices can form which one could call a "fiery wateriness." Warmth, light and air approach the plant's processes in the upper regions of its leaf life, where air is woven into watery things through the forces and activity of cosmic light; the warmth promotes and accelerates assimilation. However, in contrast to what is going on in earth and water, centrifugal tendencies already live in the finer gaseous materials that stream into the plant organization from outside and that are largely withdrawn from forces of gravity. If they are taken hold of by warmth's activity in the formation of substances, one get the formation of volatile, combustible "fiery airy" aromatic substances, essential oils. Hydrogen, the fieriest gas and the element that is the most closely related to warmth is particularly involved in their formation. The hotter the climate is the more of such essential oils one will get.

We have the highest stage of plant life in fruiting, ripening and seed formation, and warmth is the most important element. It now creates material imprints for itself in fatty oils, and no longer stimulates and promotes, and raises more and more material things into the warmth sphere. One could call essential oils substances that have become warmth, and fatty oil warmth that has become substance.

Rudolf Steiner repeatedly described seed formation along the following lines. He said that the plant was creating a space for itself in the seed, that can open itself entirely to the cosmos, and namely towards the directions from which the spiritual archetype of the particular plant species works. The way that this happens is that the protein in the seed cells is made chaotic through its "fertilization" (although this is quite different from animal fertilization). The cosmos can now intervene in this condition that has become chaotic and indeterminate, in a formative and determining way. The plant is a terrestrial cosmic being that has become too earthy through the course of its life, and it rejuvenates itself in its seed formation as it strips off its earthly ties as much as possible, and devotes itself entirely to cosmic things. The seed is a cosmic enclave in the plant. Purified and rejuvenated by the cosmos in this way, it can enter into a new connection with earthly things the next year, after the seeds have had their rest.

The formation of fatty oils also occurs through this creation of a cosmic enclave and a closing off from the earth's forces. The hydrogen process is involved a great deal here. (For example, stearic acid, one of the most common fatty acids, has the empirical formula $C_{18}H_{36}O_2$. Note that 36 of the 56 parts of this compound are hydrogen.) Since hydrogen is more related to warmth than any other earthly substance, fatty oils are able to develop warmth to a particularly high degree. (Burning 1 kg oil develops 9000 calories, and this could warm up 9 tons of water by 1 degree.)

Plant life must always oscillate between the two poles of becoming and passing out of physical existence. As Goethe also said about water, it comes from heaven, it rises to heaven, and it has to come back to earth, eternally changing.

The elements carbon and oxygen help it to come down and become earthly and to become incorporated, whereas hydrogen helps it to become cosmic and to be led back into chaos.

Why are the essential oils so volatile whereas the fatty oils are not? The essential oils are striving towards the cosmos, whereas the fatty oils have found a cosmic enclave in the plant. They have already attained their goal. In the rhythmic play between expansion and contraction in which the individual parts of the plant shape arise, the formation of essential oils belongs to the expansion of the flowers, and that of fatty oils to the contraction of the seed and germ. The former tries to volatilize in warmth; the latter tries to condense warmth in them.

One can look upon fatty oils as things that are between carbohydrates and hydrocarbons. The former arise in plants in the primal plant formation process, where water from the earth and carbon dioxide from the air condense into starch in the green leaf under the influence of light in a wonderful balance between earthly and cosmic forces. The basic carbon skeleton that supports the plant's shape is cellulose, another form of starch, whereas sugars are present in the sap that runs through it. The hydrogen and oxygen in carbohydrates are in the same 2 to 1 ratio that one finds in water. Thus they are compounds that remain close to the general biological element water, which is open to both cosmos and earth. On the other hand, hydrocarbons have ejected oxygen, and they are withdrawn from earthy conditions. Carbon is only interacting with hydrogen in them. The whole range of ways in which hydrogen and carbon can interact can be seen in the formation of petroleum in nature. The components of gasoline have the most hydrogen, such as methane, ethane and ethylene are gases that are very similar to hydrogen. Then one has the more volatile and aromatic fluidic fractions that still contain mostly hydrogen, but more carbon, as in gasoline. However the more carbon that is in the hydrocarbons, the heavier and less volatile they get, until they condense into chemically inert, solid paraffins.

The fats are in between these two poles since they seem to be connected with each of them through their inner chemical makeup, for every fat consists of glycerol and fatty acids, and is therefore built upon a polar way itself. One can separate these two poles through the saponification process.

Chemically speaking, glycerol or glycerin is a trihydroxy alcohol that is common to all fats and fatty oils. Alcohols are the first stage of combustion that results when a hydrocarbon is attacked by oxygen. In their chemical structure they are a kind of a "semi water", for water is H–OH, and methyl alcohol, for instance, CH_3OH. A hydrocarbon fragment, methyl or CH_3, has replaced a hydrogen here. Glycerin has the structural formula* $HO\ CH_2 - CH\ (OH) - OH\ CH_2$, which can be derived from the hydrocarbon propane or $CH_3–CH_2–CH_3$.

```
*  CH₂-OH                          CH₃
   |              which can be      |
   CH-OH          derived from     CH₂
   |              propane           |
   CH₂-OH                          CH₃
```

Thus it has three hydroxide or alcohol groups built into it, and it can be made from propane, a hydrocarbon with three carbons. Such alcohols belong half to water and half to hydrocarbons. Every alcohol can combine with acids to form esters, and so the trihydroxy glycerol can form a triple ester. Compounds of glycerin with three different fatty acids are our natural fats.

Glycerin's chemical makeup makes it similar to sugars, it is formed when the latter are fermented, and it tastes sweet. It is a thick, oily fluid, similar to a syrup, that has a fairly low melting point (18° C) and a high boiling point (ca 290° C) and it is characteristically liquid. Glycerol dissolves in water very easily, attracts it greedily and holds on to it, and it is therefore added to thickening agents and genes to keep them moist. It easily dissolves cooking salt and other salts and thereby reveals the water side of its constitution, and it reveals its alcohol nature through the fact that it dissolves iodine, sulfur and phosphorus. It has a phlegmatic, mercurial nature and a sluggish mobility, and it lacks intoxicating powers. Fats have a little bit of a water nature through their glycerin component, which is so important for carbohydrate formation in the assimilation process.

However, fatty acids are very close to hydrocarbons, except that they've been taken hold of by a little oxygen. Aside from the lowest members such as butyric acid, they are mostly solid, wax-like substances although Oleic acid is a thickish fluid above $60°F$. They are insoluble in water but easily soluble in ether, benzene and other sulfuric, fire related substances. As we already mentioned, the various kinds of fat and oil can be distinguished chemically by the different fatty acids they contain. Thus the specific way in which a plant is taken hold of by warmth and therewith by the hydrogen process, and is driven into the formation of seeds and maturation is expressed in the nature of the fatty acids. This occurs in a different way in spurges than in labiates, composites or palms, and castor oil correspondingly differs from marjoram seed oil, sunflower oil and coconut oil.

In evaluating a plant fat one always has to consider the whole plant process, and not just the chemical analysis. Unadulterated olive oil is a particularly fine oil through the nature of the whole olive process and the hard earth nature in it has been purified into the grace and peace of the sun's life. One used to calm stormy waves with it, one lit up one's evenings with the mild light of an oil lamp, and one never poured oil onto a fire. Olive oil gave some body to foods and its mildness was used to offset sharp, sour and salty things, and a thin layer of it helped to keep one's warmth organization together through daily massages. Such a protective sheath is important, since warmth is the carrier of man's being or I. Olive oil became a foundation for healing ointments when combined with beeswax and worked in with some medicinal herbs or extracted them with it, as one directed their power into the body from outside through the skin organ in this way. It is still being used today, and the olive tree that gives us so much will no doubt remain a benevolent companion of human life far into the future.

*

The Dogbane Family - Apocynaceae

There is one form of plant existence that is rare in our temperate zone, although it is often seen in tropical forests, and that is vines and creepers that seem to go on almost endlessly. The wild grapes, ivy and clematis that we have in our woods are about the only examples of this. Bind weeds, beans and bryony are only puny imitations of the up to 100 m long rope stems as thick as one's arm that wind, hang and swing from the tree tops in the tropics, and such vines belong to quite a large variety of plant families. Goethe pointed to the two principles that govern plant growth, the vertical tendency, that becomes manifest in the upright growth of a tree or stem, and the spiral tendency that one can see in the serpentine arrangement of leaves around an upright stem. Some plants lack the ability to grow this firm staff in the middle, and they have an excessive spiral tendency that takes hold of and transforms the shoot, side shoots, leaves or inflorescence, so that the whole stem winds up another upright plant or else about its leaves, side shoots or inflorescence that have been transformed into tendrils help the plant to raise itself. It is not a matter of cleverly thought out adaptations and mechanisms in a "struggle for existence" here, but of the one–sided and therefore striking emergence of a formative principle that is inherent in all plants, including the nonwinding varieties. Winding plants lack the solar axis or the line of forces between the sun and the center of the earth, along which the cosmic plant I works, as we explained in Volume I. The planets that wind around the sun's path with spiral loops give the plant's body of formative forces the impulse to arrange leaf growth in a spiral manner. The ancient peoples looked upon Mercury as both a physical planet and divine, spiritual beings who live in it, and it especially reveals itself in the winding of leaves around something, so that one could say that the sign it wields here is a plant caduceus.

The relatives of many plants that we only know as herbs in our latitudes become trees in the tropics. The vertical tendency becomes mightier there and the earth projects up into the heights as gigantic trunks. The one sided spiral tendency also becomes very manifest in the vines that continue to wind upwards and onwards endlessly. A proper earthly plant exists in a vertical position; it is devoted to gravity below and to anti–gravity or cosmic levity above. A vine or creeper cannot overcome gravity through its own power; it would have to creep over the earth like an animal in the direction of its backbone if it didn't find another, upright plant that replaced the missing upright. Just as a snake in the animal kingdom is an excessive backbone process with no limbs to lift it away from the ground, and therefore it is more bound to gravity than other animals, so a vine in the plant kingdom, that puts out one node and leaf after another, just as a snake has one vertebra after another, is unable to get away from gravity by itself.

The lower elements, forest humus and ground moisture, are readily available to vines; they suck in a lot of moisture, and if one hits some of them with a machete they give out drinkable water, like plant springs. Rubber plants and many other species are full of milky juices, and some of them are even potable. The broiling, damp, tropical heat promotes vines' growth. Light doesn't get down to the jungle's floor much because it is filtered and weakened by the many green leaves. But once a vine gets up to the top branches and the crown of leaves, it encounters its astral region and it arrives at its flowering process which often takes hold of it in a mighty way and give it large funnels, many racemes, beautiful colors, powerful aromas. The flowering process sometimes overpowers the etheric body that has been exhausted by the rhythmic stem and leaf process so that poisons can form.

A large number of the 1,000 species of Apocynocea are vines and creepers and many of them form milky juices. However, this plastic, fluid element can easily become congested. Thickened branches can form that swell up like cactuses. Species that grow more out in the open and can grow into small trees form thick, soft, crabby trunks or ones that are shaped like a sugarloaf. One sometimes finds glands that excrete fluids in their leaf axils. Nectar drips out of the blossoms, many species have juicy berries and some of them are even edible. Lacmellia edulis is a small tree in Columbia with potable, milky juice and edible sweet cherries (lac = milk, mel = honey).

Apocynoceae leaves are plastic and roundish, never pinnate or divided, and formed more by water than by air.

Although a few species have berries, most develop a bipartite pad or capsule out of an ovary that is always inferior; the pad pops open when it is ripe and releases many tufted or winged seeds into the wind and thus does after all conquer air and levity.

Many species form very poisonous glycosides or alkaloids in their milky sap, wood and bark (ouabain in Acocanthera species, serpentine in Rauwolfia, strophanthidin in strophanthus, and conessine in periwinkle.)

It is easy to see why if one considers how strong the vital forces are that take hold of cosmic astrality, but can't break through. Since these poisons usually paralyze the heart very quickly, the natives in tropical Asia, Africa and South America have put them on their arrow heads since time immemorial for rapid killing action.

One would expect dog banes to have a curative effect in cases where the astral body has pressed into the etheric part of the human rhythmic system in an unhealthy way, since their strong flowering process discloses a pressing in of the astral region into a hypertrophic rhythmic system. If the human fluid organization is not permeated by etheric forces enough, the wrestling of the plant process with the force of gravity, especially in the fluidic organization, will add invigoration and levity to the curative effect. One finds heart stimulants in this family that are somewhat similar to those in cactuses and spurges, although the tendency to form vines adds another dimension.

The only dog banes we have in our latitudes are hemp dogbane, oleander, and the greater and lesser periwinkles. The latter are such modest plants with evergreen leaves in stems that creep through rocky woods that one can hardly believe that they belong to a family that has such powerful growth forces. The following is a brief description of the important medicinal plants rauwolfia, strophanthus, nerium oleander and hemp dogbane.

Apocynum cannabinum – Hemp Dogbane (Cascadia Hemp)

This perennial with branching stems grows 3–5 feet tall from various places on a rampant, thick root stock into the realm of air, and light. It emphasizes a linear tendency right into the plainly drawn ribs of its pointed, lanceolate, smooth edged leaves, and thereby points to the creeping vine nature of this family above ground and not just in the rootstock that meanders underground. This linear striving is also reflected in the formation of many fibers in the rootstock and stems which give the plant its "hemp" dogbone name. The stem and the side branches terminate their linear striving in bright, white delicate inflorescence that bear clusters of tubular little, five pointed flowers. Long pods release silky, tufted seeds.

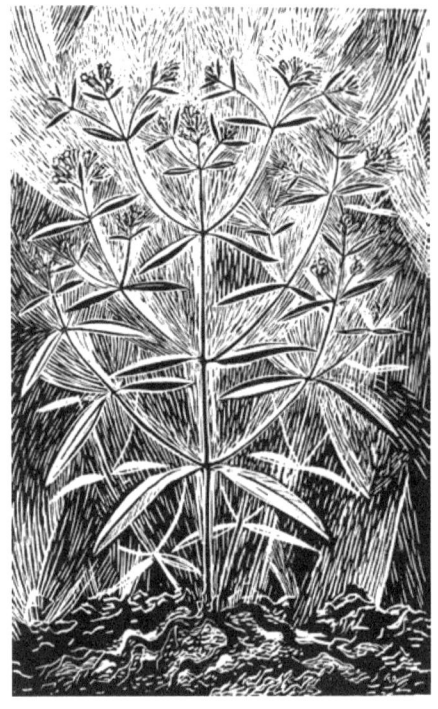

Hemp dogbane sketches on insignia for itself in the visible world, out of a plastic, fluidic root filled with milky juice and through a striving line into the realm of light and air that is resolutely drawn by growth. It lets itself be borne rhythmically upwards in this way through the formation of its many leaves.

Our plant leads its rampant milky root stock life up into shaping and illuminating activities. It will be able to exert formative, levitational effects upon man's fluidic organism and to stimulate shaping, excretory effects from the upper organization, especially when this fluidic organism that is insufficiently permeated by the etheric body has become too physical and sinks into earthly gravity. That is why Apocynum is used for edematous conditions due to heart disease. The plant contains cardioglycosides like those in foxgloves and so do oleander, strophanthus and a few other dogbanes. (Refer to section on Digitalis.)

Nerium Oleander – Oleander

Oleander or Rose Bay is a shrub or small tree that grows along rivers in the Mediterranean and Middle East regions, just as willows grow along our brooks. It sends its roots into moist ground and its slender rods with their many whorls of three, narrow, evergreen laurel-like leaves into the double light that comes from above and that is reflected from water. The watery element changes into a milky juice that courses through the whole shrub. Hydrophilia intensifies into photophilia and thermophilia as the plant rises out of the subterranean realm into the air and the region of the upper formative forces. And when the oleander breaks out into its many pink and red flowers in summer and fills the evening air with its intoxicating, volatile, sweet aroma, one gladly admits that it has combined the stern character of a laurel bay with the grace of roses. It is considered one of the most beautiful plants in its zone.

However, the red is too inflammatory, there are too many flowers. Oleander's soul sphere or astral region takes hold of its vital processes too strongly. The chastity of rose buds is missing, and one can literally see the toxin forming excess, but only enough to form cardio glycosides that are similar to those in digitalis and not enough to form alkaloids that contain nitrogen, as in poppies. The excessive astral impulse presses into the etheric, fluidic system but is unable to punch through it and to break into and disintegrate the physical protein and to let its fragments appear in the formation of alkaloids. Nevertheless, oleander is quite poisonous, and even the honey that bees make from its nectar is considered to be dangerous.

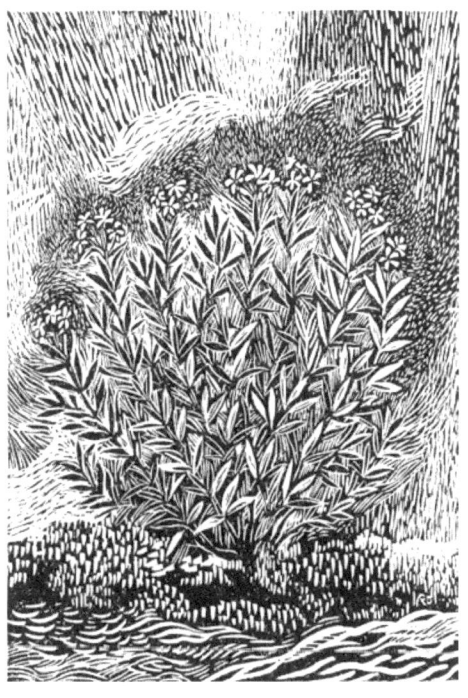

One can see the typical characteristics of the family in its tufted seeds and great vitality. Any twigs cut from it and stuck in the ground will quickly take root. The winding of vines is overcome here and the power to stand erect has been attained.

The healing effect of its leaves and flowers is felt between the rhythmic and metabolic systems, and they regulate the intervention of the astral body in the etheric body in this region. Its effect on the heart is well known and will be discussed more in the following.

Strophanthus Species

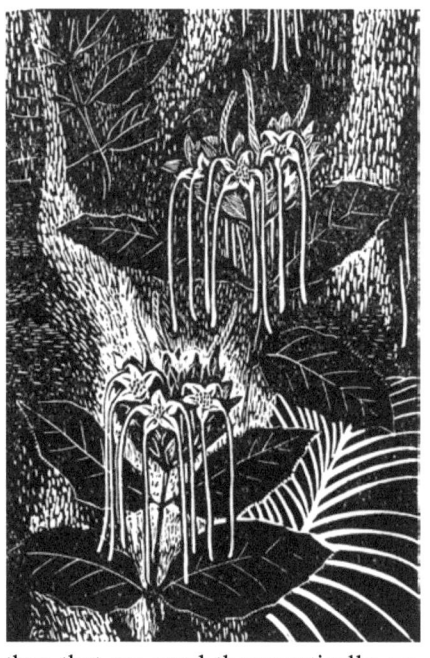

Over 40 species of strophanthus are spread out between West Africa and East Asia, and they are all more or less vines. The genus gets its name from its long flower buds that look like spirally twisted ropes. The whole dogbane family lets the spiral tendency of its winding, looping growth fade out in the spiral rotation of the petals in the flower buds. The opened flowers of some dogbanes love the shape of a pinwheel that seems to be rotating slightly, due to the asymmetrical petals. One can see this particularly well in the periwinkle that grows in woods, but also in oleander flowers.

The three species of strophanthus that are used therapeutically are vines or clambering shrubs in West and East Africa. Strophanthus Kombe, S. gratus and S. hispidus climb up medium to tall size trees in a battle between gravity and levity. The evergreen leaves are thick, elliptical, hairy, undivided and opposite. After growth seems to have continued long enough, they bear terminal clusters of spirally twisted flower buds that are stuck on like candles, which stand up freely in spite of their length, as if they were being pulled up by a rotating stream of air, mocking gravity like a pirouette in ballet. However, once these bright colored flowers open, the long tails at the tips of the flower petals fall down limply under the force of gravity. The longitudinal growth that was temporarily paralyzed by the flowering impulse now shoots mightily into the ovaries and drives two carpel leaves that are held together by the stigma ring but are otherwise free, 8–12 inches out from the receptacle. But when the stigma dies the carpels split apart and sink down into a horizontal position. The long capsules burst and release many tufted seeds into the air. So after a lot of back and forth everything eventually dissolves into air, light and levity.

The wrestling of gravity and levity forces has found its most perfect imprint in hydrogen, and therefore it is permissible to call it a hydrogen process. See the discussion about medicinal plants for meteorological organs,[28] especially the section about medicinal plants for the heart, for more details. Rudolf Steiner gave some interesting indications about the relationship between the hydrogen and heart processes. He indicated strophanthus seeds as a starting point for remedies that could be used to counteract disturbances of rhythms in our time. However, he recommended that one should use its fatty seed oil for this, whereas medicine mainly uses the pure glycosides that have been isolated and crystallized from strophanthus seeds.

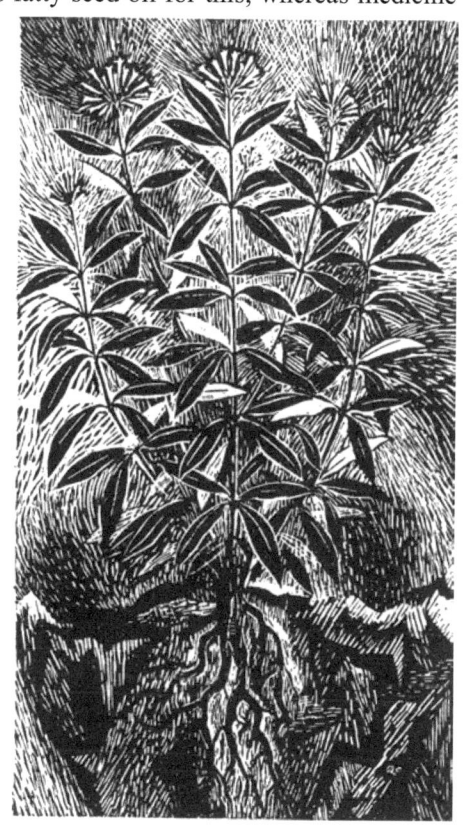

African hunters use the strongly poisonous nature of the dried out, milky juice and other parts of the winding plant in the form of a very effective arrow poison.

Rauwolfia serpentina

Rauwolfia canescens and R. serpentina were used in ancient oriental medicine out of a total of over 130 species, and they have also come to the attention of western medicine.

Rauwolfia grows to about 3 feet high half way up India's mountains. It bears whorls of three or four

---

[28] See the section on typical properties of medicinal plants for the liver, kidneys, lungs and heart.

lanceolate, smooth edged leaves, dark green above, along stems with white bark that are crowned at the end by clusters of flower buds. The latter eventually open into many white or red delicate flowers with long tubes that are slightly inflated in the middle, with five points. After they fade the peduncles continue to grow, and carries small, black pitted fruits a few inches higher.

The deeply indented flowers and the plant's rather scrubby size, compared with other milky dogbanes, enables one to see that there must be a vigorous working of astral forces into the life processes with the formation of alkaloid poisons rather than the glycosides that were present in the other dogbanes already discussed. It produces a certain loosening of the human astral body, its normal connection with the physical world is dampened and abnormal, and hallucinations take its place. That is why people in India treated certain kinds of "mental diseases" with it. In western medicine, its bitter root is often used to lower blood pressure.

The intensity of the astral body's intervention in the rhythmic system, and especially in the circulating action, becomes manifest in blood pressure. However, if one drastically reduces the abnormally high blood pressure of a sclerotic, for instance, one is only eliminating a symptom temporarily and is not bringing about a real healing. Western psychiatrists looked at the tranquilizing effect of the drugs in the root and hoped that they had found a real psychotherapeutic drug in them.

*

THE HEATHER FAMILY – ERICACEAE

Northern Fruits

The Ericacea being likes an interaction with light, moisture and coolness, whether it is found in moors, bogs, high mountain or the polar regions in Europe. Asia and the Americas, and its 1350 species are spread around. Cosmic forces predominate over weakened earth forces in such regions. Granites and other primal siliceous rocks that are related to light tend to be present there. (Silica is a kind of a mineralized light). The plants are strongly formed, well built, tough, lignified, perennial and are often small and slow growers, although the strawberry tree and other escapees into warmer regions are larger. The evergreen, undivided leaves that are often contracted into something almost like needles are reminiscent of conifers. Some species constitute the underbrush in well lighted forests.

They do not lose themselves in rampant growth but they hold their own fluidic organization together in a strict way in the midst of much moisture, and even in swamps and moors. There are a number of things that keep their fluids from evaporating into the air. Their roots live with fungal material that spins around and permeates them, and that would like to produce a semi-living substratum for them in well watered soil with hardly any minerals. This is reminiscent of the three kingdoms of nature on the old Moon that we have mentioned several times in this book, and especially of the half living, lowest mineral plant kingdom that partly consisted of something like wood, but contained no minerals.

Heather plants grow up in such an environment like miniature trees, and their spiraling or opposite leaves do not change much as they go up the stem. They bunch together into dense rosettes at the end of the shoots and pass over into a colorful and fragrant flowering process with wide open, rayed, flower funnels, in which a strong sugar process flows out as nectar that bees love. Or else the flowering process sinks deep into the stem and leaf region, in which case one gets nodding flower jugs, inferior ovaries that are devoted to the germinal growth forces for the root, leaf and stem region and that swell up into juicy, sweet berry fruits. (The fruits of the first kind are dry and the seeds are light and sometimes winged, here light, air and warmth were the dominant forces.) Thus Ericaceae have an active sugar process that remains permeated by strong formative forces, which one perceives in the somewhat tart taste of their fruits. We have in this family huckleberry, cranberry, bear berry, mountain cranberry, bog berry, crow berry and other fruits of the far north and of the high mountains.

Earth evolution repeated the Old Moon evolution in the Lemurian epoch,[29] and it brought an essentially new creative impulse into earth existence in the following Atlantean epoch. The plants on old Moon became the higher plants on earth via this evolutionary path. The half living, moors became terra firma, the formative tendencies in root and stem became realized, the foggy air became filled with light and vegetation responded to cosmic forces that penetrated ever deeper through the formation of real flowers. (Lemurian plants were still more like gigantic, floating, swimming algae in a dense primal atmosphere. See Volume I

---

[29] See the chapter on World Evolution and the Human Being in Rudolf Steiner's *Occult Science, an Outline*

and the section on lower plants in this volume.) The Atlantean epoch ended with the Ice Age, and the sinking of the Atlantean continent was accompanied by the subsequent melting of huge glacial areas (the flood). Ericaceae bear the traces of this evolution in their characteristics. The damp and cold, gigantic moor lands that the melting glacial regions left behind corresponded to the slow, inhibited growth of lower shrubs. The air that had become clear, transparent and filled with light permitted this growth to pass over into the beautiful variety of colors in an active formation of flowers. The Ericaceae that looked like rhododendron arose, with more and more species as one goes towards the East, from our Alpine roses to the azaleas of the Eastern Asiatic mountains. The cosmic flowering process is sucked up more by the shoot from the earth or by the stem and leaf principle in huckleberries and other vacciniums that bear berries. The flowers sink down into gravity and become distributed along the axis of the stems rather than bunching up into magnificent terminal clusters. The ovaries became inferior, and earth and water forces make the berries swell up. Members of the third subfamily or heather, grow on siliceous, sandy, dry heaths, and emphasize a linear striving of leaves and flowers along the stem, somewhat as conifers do. The Ericacea type is able to put its imprint upon whole landscapes and to give them a basic mood of seriousness and longing.

The characteristics of our plant family become manifest in the substances that the metabolism of its individual members form, and not just in their shapes. They contain a lot of tannins which is characteristic for plants that bear the forces of the astral sphere into the etheric organization particularly strongly, and thereby develop an intensive flowering process. We already spoke of their strong sugar forming processes; added to these are glycoquinines which can regulate the sugar metabolism in a curative way in diabetics and other patients. The brooding, moist warmth over moors stimulates the formation of dully aromatic essential oils (as in wild rosemary and winter green). Plants that live in damp cold and that intensively incorporate the air and light of atmospheric life together with astralization processes as a counterpole form salicylic acid compounds (see Meadowsweet in Volume 1, and Willows in Volume 2). A very strong flowering process tends to form poisonous plants and there is something narcotic about the formation of nectar in certain species of rhododendron.

The healing virtue of the Ericaceae is in their capacity to combat inflammations from colds, rheumatic diseases and gout, and chills in the fluidic organization. We will say more about this in the following descriptions of the most useful medicinal plants in this family.

Ledum palustre – *Marsh Rosemary*

On moors we encounter this small, evergreen, woody, ramified shrub with its leathery, linear leaves that are glossy green above, rusty red below, and curled under at the edges. The many terminal clusters of white, intoxicating inflorescences open in May and June. Even the leaves and branches smell resinous, sensuous, aromatic, intoxicating, sweetish and acrid at the same time. The watery element becomes ignited by the sultry heat on the damp moors in summer; it steams and glows at the same time. Much nectar flows from the receptacles.

Wild rosemary grows on northern peat bogs in Europe, Asia and America up to and beyond the 70 degree line. The northern, cold winters belong to it just as the long summer days with their abundance of light and their sultry boggy atmosphere.

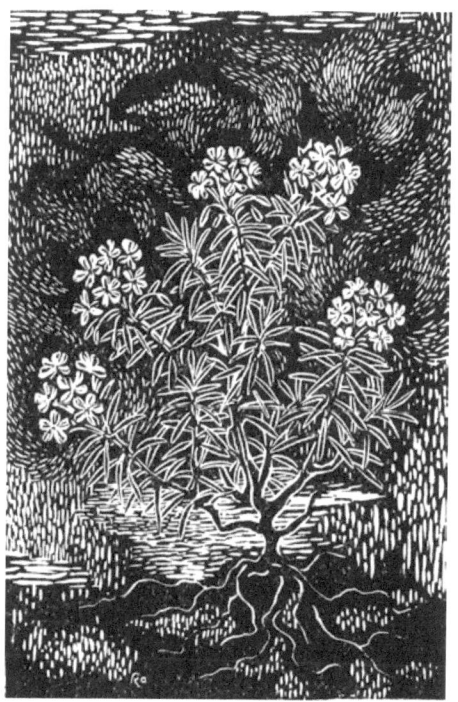

The whole plant, especially the flowers and leaves, is full of the essential oil ledol that has stimulating and intoxicating effects. It also contains arbutin, a flavon glycoside, and some tannins. (See the description of Bearberry below for more details.)

From the many previous discussions of strong flowering processes in plants in this book, the reader will already be aware that one can mainly expect effects upon the metabolic system from this plant. Weakened warmth and I organizations that tend to contract chronic colds don't carry out metabolic processes sufficiently, and they don't give their building up action an impulse that leads to a fully human body. What comes from food is not completely divested of its foreign character. Since the I organization intervenes too weakly, the astral organization begins to work too strongly. It brings about degradation and excretion in the organism in a disorderly way at places where no organs are prepared to take in and excrete what has been separated. The organism responds to such activities with inflammatory processes. Plants that grow around moors, and especially ones like ledum can address the abnormal interaction of man's members that underlie this kind of pathological, rheumatic conditions.

Kalmia latifolia – Mountain Laurel

Kalmia is an evergreen shrub with laurel leaves that grow 4 to 10 feet high on the boggy, sour soils of eastern North America. Compared with wild rosemary, it lacks the aromatic element, and the many pink flowers are pulled into the leaf and stem region more strongly. The plant lives in the leaf process much more strongly than wild rosemary does.

Its healing effect on inflammatory, rheumatic processes is therefore displaced more towards the rhythmic system. Mountain laurel is especially indicated for such diseases if the heart is involved.

Rhododendron ferrugineum – The Rust–leafed Alpine Rose

This "alpine rapture" covers the rocky, gravelly slopes and waste lands of the Alps from the edge of the forest up to rock niches at 3000 meters. The strong, springy, brownish branches and the shiny, evergreen leaves that are rust colored underneath make the knee high shrub into a heartwarming sight in the desolate rocky wastelands of the central Alps and in the gloomy primal schist mountains, especially in early summer when extensive slopes and whole plateaus are glowing in a pink rapture of marvelous flowers.

Its branches first pass over into bunches of oblong, lanceolate leaves with resinous glands and then into luxuriant clusters of funnel form companulate flowers that contain a lot of nectar. Tiny seeds in the capsules are scattered by the wind. The Ericaceae get their necessary moisture from the foggy air and snow, and a sod like soil or damp humus forms around their roots.

This plant is a characteristic, common plant in the places where it grows, and Rudolf Steiner indicated its use as a basic remedy for the inhabitants of those regions in order to combat the frequently melancholic nature of the life forces organizations there.

Like many other Ericaceae, the plant has been used for rheumatism, gout and inflammatory diseases of the male genital tract.

Arctostaphylos Uva ursi – Bearberry

Bearberry covers dry, loose, warm soils with a dense carpet of creeping stems, as an undergrowth in illuminated pine forests far up into the north, and it loves the shade of bushes in the mountains. Therewith our plant deviates from the other Ericaceae we looked at, which like boggy soil. Its short branches with bunches of fleshy, evergreen, obovate leaves bend upwards and bear small clusters of terminal flowers. The pinkish white, hanging, urn-shaped flowers that open up a little in their tips contain a lot of nectar, and they open in the spring. Compared with huckleberries, cowberries and cranberries, our red berries are mealy and dry rather than juicy, and they usually contain five stone 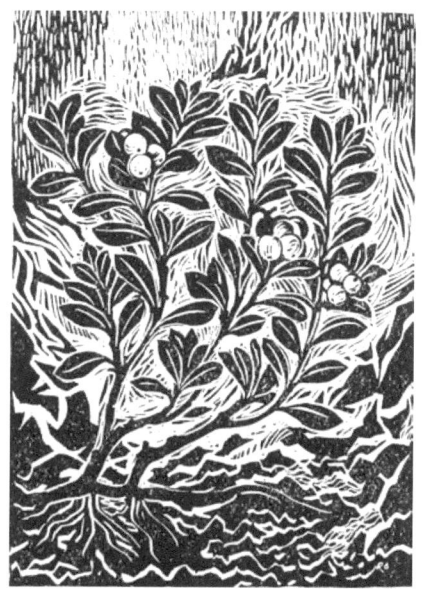 pits. Their ovaries are superior, contrary to the other species we looked at.

The leaves that are gathered and dried in the early fall have healing forces. In addition to the essential oils and tannins that are generally found in Ericaceae, these leaves contain arbutoside and methyl or hydroquinone and methyl hydroquinone that are bound to glucose. (They are also found in other Erica leaves, pear leaves and in Bergenia grassifolia, all of which contain a lot of tannins.)

These phenols with two hydroxide groups that thirst for oxygen point to a process by means of which our plant would like to draw the airy region into itself. The strong disinfectant properties of all phenols point to

221

processes here that dampen life and don't leave lower, parasitic life any room. This and their proximity to tannins point to processes between the astral and etheric and the airy and fluidic organizations. Rudolf Steiner once said that phenol has a paralyzing effect upon the astral body. The kidney bladder tract is an organ region in which the astral body organizes the fluidic system in an especially active way as it builds things up towards the interior and excretes things outwardly. Preparations made from bearberry leaves tend to alleviate conditions where the lawfulness of the inorganic world pushes into the excretory process too early and too strongly, as one can see from the formation of stones and from decomposition and rotting processes that should only be connected with urine outside the body.

Vaccinium Myrtillus – Huckleberry, Bilberry

Huckleberry shrubs are known to every one, so that a detailed description is unnecessary here. This plant likes damp soils with a lot of humus that are moderately shaded by trees or shrubs. It creates a sour humus for itself with a lot of silica but little limestone. The bluish blackberry develops a lot of sugar, acid and tannin, and it has a salutory effect on the gastro-intestinal tract. We already mentioned that glucoquinines lower the sugar level in blood; their presence in its leaves (which produce sugar) make it a good tea to use in the treatment of diabetes. Since they also contain some arbutin, they are used for bladder ailments, just as bearberry leaves are.

Vaccinium vitis–idaea –
Cowberry, Mountain Cranberry

Cowberry or mountain cranberry grows in about the same places as huckleberry does, in northern America, Europe and Asia. It loves moor lands, heaths and siliceous soils, and it turns towards the light much more strongly than huckleberries do. Its small shiny, leathery, evergreen leaves are also better formed and more delicate that those in its sister that likes shady areas more. The noble, northern fruit grows particularly well in Finland with its granite domes, damp sea landscapes in between, and long, luminous summer days. (Up to now, people have considered southern fruit to be particularly valuable; it is about time to bring out the different but equally great advantages of berry fruits from the north by using the corresponding term, a "northern fruit").

Like bearberry, cowberry leaves contain the arbutin that inhibits rotting and fermentation, and the tasty, spicy, red berries contain many fruit acids, Vitamins A and C, sugar, and benzoic acid, the very substance that the chemical industry gives our housewives to use as a preservative, but which is prepared by nature here in a small dose, so that it has no harmful effects.

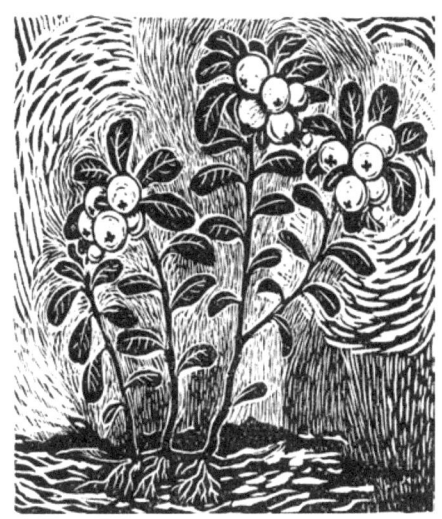

In a way cowberries are the greatest contrast to grapes, for the latter tend to ferment most easily, whereas the former are the hardest to ferment. Finnish cowberries are pounded in vats until they are swimming in their own juice and then traded. The resulting sauce keeps very well, and it helps one to digest wild game, roast goose and cheese fare. It has a stimulating and ordering effect upon the digestive process, and its blend of sweet, sour and crudely aromatic substances stimulate the I and astral body to break down more food as a preliminary stage for the subsequent build up in the digestive organs. Cowberry's ability to suppress sugar fermentation comes to meet the activity that the I has to carry out in connection with the sugar processes inside the body and especially in the head organization. In a certain respect sugar is the substance in man that carries the I. It must not ferment even to the slightest extent, especially in the sensory, nervous system.[30] Cowberry sugar has been elaborated by nature in such a way that it comes to meet this striving. This helps one to understand why Rudolf Steiner recommended a remedy that was prepared from cowberries for headache in children.

---

[30] See the chapter about grape vine plants.

PRIMROSES – PRIMULACEAE
Plants with Etheric Vernal Rhythms
Saponins, Salicylic Acids

The supersensible force structure that can be looked upon as the Primulaceae type exposes its nature in space and time in such a way that it becomes manifest in a rhythmic transition and a balance between two principles, cosmic powers and terrestrial processes that loosen themselves from consolidation and rigidification. For the best spatial and temporal conditions for the various primroses are the northern parts of the temperate zones and their mountains, and the transition from wintry to vernal earth processes. Their 600 species unfold between the "head and chest processes" of the earth organism.[31]

Some members of this family love to latch onto the ground firmly with root stocks and to creep through it, or to feel their way along its surface with creeping stems and offshoots. The mostly deciduous leaves like to remain on the ground as a rosette, even when the plant grows and closes off its long straight shoots with a circular motion. Primroses' slender flower stalks usually shoot up from the ground and carry up clusters or racemes of beautiful flower buds. The funnel form or long tubular flowers that spread out radially show off their clear colors and delicate, refreshing scents. The calyxes often surround a good portion of these flowers and sometimes become inflated, and like the flowers they have a long life. The ovary is usually above the base of the petals; it doesn't sink into the stem, and it thereby tells us that it is more devoted to cosmic activities than to earthly ones. The fruit dries out into an airy capsule.

This is the basic shape of this family; it has all of the characteristics of plants that grow high up in the mountains. A strong development of the poles and a weak manifestation of the rhythmic center is the signature of vernal plants and of plants that grow on high mountains. They bring their flowers up out of the roots almost directly. The leaves that develop in spring do not get crowned with flowers in the summer or fall, but the

---

[31] One can look upon the earth as a gigantic, threefold organism that has its metabolic part in the tropics, its head part at the poles and its rhythmic organization in the temperate zones, as we have pointed out before.

flowers' germs first go down into the roots and are borne by the wintry, cosmic world. The primrose being incarnates into such polar tensions.

The delicate, nodding, reddish violet or bluish soldanella flowers bare directly through the snow. The tiny, dark green leaves, like those of cyclamen, only unfold after the snow has melted. The well over 200 species of primulas come next, as the largest part of the family, and also the rock jasmines (androsaceae) with their 90 species. They come up at the beginning of spring after the snow has left, earlier in the lowlands and later in the mountains. There are a lot of them in the Alps, Caucasus, Himalayas and in Chinese and Japanese mountains, and some species go 4000 meters up. The only species in the tropics are on the peaks of the highest mountains, for instance, primula imperialis, the tiered cowslip in Java, and Mt. Sinai has its own species. In the subtropics the growth that is held up in the rootstock in our climes pushes upwards in a luxuriant way and brings about the formation of tiers in the inflorescence, that is, growth continues through the cluster of flowers and produces more clusters further on.

Once spring has passed, the primrose species that come out then keep on looking for vernal situations such as cool, damp banks of lakes, seas and rivers, damp, shady ditches and openings in woods. They appear as species of lysimachia (garden loosestrife, moneywort), and chickweed wintergreen; water lily swims without roots in dead river arms, and it lifts itself over the water out of submerged whorls of leaves with long peduncles or scopes on pink flowers with yellow throats. Scarlet pimpernel grows in vegetable beds and in the moist shade of grain fields, and its flowers open in the morning sun. The sea milkwort (Glaux) with its thick leaves, and common brookweed (Samolus) grow along the seashore. These species that unfold at the beginning of summer send up leafy shoots, and therewith try to become bushes. That is how certain Lysimachias in the Mediterranean look, they have clusters of thyme-like flowers. However, the type doesn't take enough earth forces into itself to really become a shrub or a tree.

As the days get shorter again, fall begins and cyclamen opens up its pink buds, the flowers nod down to the earth that is closing itself off, and end the primrose cycle with a similar gesture to the one with which the soldanelles began it in the spring.

The etheric signature of cowslip or key of heaven is to mix into the life processes elements that are working in the spring air's moving breath and in the sunlight that is radiating in from the Aries region, and that are living in the water that is freed from its solid state and in the earth that is permeated by resurrection forces. Such an interweaving gives rise to the saponins that are present in almost all cowslips. Their material properties are like a rigidified copy of the dynamics of the forces and processes that we just described. If one dissolves a saponin in some water and shakes it, one gets a nice head of foam. The airy element is closely connected with water in the foam formation. The water forms a lot of little air bubbles. The watery element breathes in air with the aid of saponins. If one adds a solution that contains traces of saponins to a blood preparation, it immediately dissolves the blood corpuscles, and the red dye in them separates from the blood's proteins (hemolysis). However, the air's oxygen connects itself with the fluid blood in the lung's alveoli through the dye in the blood.

Another property of saponins is that they act like strong poisons upon fish; they paralyze and injure the gills through which fish get the oxygen that is dissolved in water into their blood. Native catch a lot of fish with the aid of crushed plants that contain saponins, albeit not in a very sportsman like way.

The main curative effect of saponins is upon the intestinal and lung regions. In the intestines they promote the passage of chyle into the lymph vessels, which it enters as very fine droplets. This is a sphere of activity in the organism where mercury, that likes to break up into droplets so much, is particularly active in as a process and a remedy. Here the broken down food is taken up into the realm of bodily fluids and the etheric body, so that it can be led towards the cardiopulmonary process and therewith can be permeated with air and vitalized. This is a second mercurial region in which saponins can exert their influence. They promote expectoration when the lungs fill with mucous during colds and they facilitate the entry of air into the blood.

Still, a third property of saponins must be mentioned: Natives often use saponins as antidotes for snake poisons. The latter inhibit breathing and decompose the blood. The chemical structures of snake poisons and of saponins are somewhat similar; one could call the former animal sapotoxins. Inoculation with snake poisons or with the juices of plants that contain saponins confers a certain immunity against snake poisoning.

Saponins also stimulate glands to secrete. Thereby one works upon the fluidic organism via the glands. Saliva flows, digestive glands secrete more fluids, and more urine is passed. Glandular organs are mainly created by the etheric body, and therefore they are somewhat plantlike. The astral body works into them from outside, just as it does in plants, where the astral body promotes flower formation by touching the plant's etheric body from outside eliciting nectar and other fluids from the fluidic organism.

One thing that characterizes the saponins is that they don't work upon organs that mediate sensation, perception and consciousness, that is, they don't affect the senses and nerves. The latter organs in the body are ones with which the astral body has a continual connection. Saponins work upon regions where the astral rhythmically unites and separates from the etheric. This occurs in a vegetative, unconscious way. Saponins produce no consciousness phenomena. That is why they furnish no narcotics. They enter into all rhythms where the astral body works into the fluidic organization, from the glands in the metabolic region to the blood and lungs in the rhythmic system. These are mercurial processes; saponins are a vegetable mercury. Quicksilver's medical sphere of activity is surprisingly similar to that of these plant substances.

The forces that follow in the course of a year are present simultaneously in the human organism. The earth brings the interaction of its being with the cosmos to expression in the seasons. Winter brings a predominance of cosmic powers and a dampening of the earth life that is closing itself off from them; the earth is opened to all cosmic things and is connected with them in the summer; spring and fall are rhythmic, intermediate states. The earth also bears the seasons in it simultaneously, for it is always winter at the poles, summer in the tropics, and it goes through rhythmic intermediate conditions in the temperate zones. Since man is the being who harmoniously includes the cosmic and earthly worlds in his body, and can find a more cosmic, wintry region in his head with its dampened life processes and its tendency to solidify, and a summery, tropical one in the metabolic system with its warming and dissolution processes. The middle, rhythmic system expresses itself in a vernal or autumnal way, it becomes vernally enlivened in inhalation, and autumnally dampened in exhalation. Primroses connect themselves with localities (temperate zones) and seasons (spring; or fall in the cyclamens) where one has this rhythmic interaction of cosmic and earthly things that harmonize with their nature. They have a healing effect upon rhythmic processes where the airy organization that is taken hold of by the astral body enlivens and imparts rhythm to the fluidic organism that is permeated by the etheric body in a vernal way.

*

We will go into this in more detail in the following discussion of the five most important medicinal plants in this family.

Primula veris [32] – *European Cowslip, Key of Heaven*

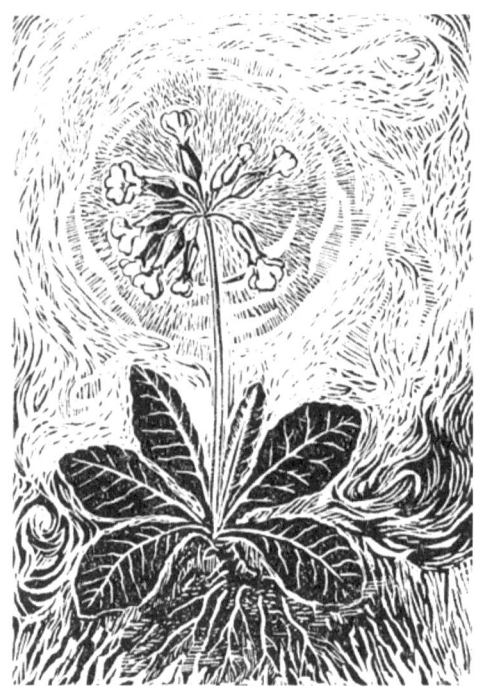

The 400 primula species are the largest part of the primrose family and Primulo veris is the representative primrose, the species that comes closest to the primal motif; it is almost the primal phenomenon of the primrose being. Its flowers really introduce spring and Eastertide in the cooler parts of the northern temperate zone, and it is at home there from China to the Atlantic. It likes well lit meadows that are still damp from the winter's moisture, but are already warmed by the Aries sun and are moved about by the stormy atmosphere: "Rise, O shining light,/ Take hold of developing beings,/Grasp the weaving of forces,/Radiate and awaken life." That's how Rudolf Steiner once characterized the nature of Aries effects in a poem that expresses the effects of the twelve zodiacal signs. (*The Twelve Moods*, Mercury Press) Key of Heaven is a messenger of this rising, an image of the stormy mixing of the elements and of the latest

---

[32] Replace P. officinalis

meeting of the cosmos and the earth. Healing forces work into earth events everywhere, winter's rigidity and congestions in life forces are overcome, Raphael, Mercury, the archangel of healing rules the hour, and blood and breath are renewed. Spring cures have been fashionable for millennia, and key of heaven is often included in these. The earth's atmosphere and circulation of fluids are renewed and invigorated. Oxygen, the tender of life's flame, rises from the greening plant world again, and fruitful rains pour down. All of this belongs to Key of Heaven, for it forms its body from such realms and such events.

It unites itself with the earth with a strong and short root stock for a number of years and spreads out a rosette of long stemmed leaves that rise from the ground somewhat, out of whose center a long scape rises rapidly, that spreads out its magnificent, shining gold cluster. The long, tubular flowers with a decorative fringe and golden red dots in their throats are surrounded by an inflated, slender calyx; they hesitantly search for an equilibrium between light levity and earth gravity and they all feel their way towards the sun and turn in its direction while half of them bow down to the ground and the rest of them raise themselves up. That's why a cowslip meadow shines most beautifully when it is looked at from the direction of the sun.

A delicate and yet powerfully refreshing scent tells one about the invigorating forces that connect themselves with the flowering process in this plant. The fruit is an airy, dry capsule, and it turns up into a strictly vertical position. The weaving of forces that becomes manifest through such forms creates a variety of material copies of itself. We already spoke about saponins. One should also mention the carotene dyes that are hidden in the green leaves but are visible in the golden flowers, and which become the vitamin A in the human organism that connects all organs that originated from the ectoderm (skin, sense organs) with nutritional and enlivening forces. Balancing, enlivening forces counteract the degradative and hardening forces that arise through the strong influence of light, as an excess of formative forces and as a solidifying silica effect in these organ regions. Carotenes mediate light forces for the chlorophyll in plants, and then help light to incarnate. The visual purple at the back of the eye that takes in the light's formative impressions as a destructive imprint, and that continuously regenerates itself from the blood, is a metamorphosis of carotene. Vitamin A deficiency makes all the organs that come from the ectoderm dry out. Carotene enlivens silica's activities, and it cushions the destructive effects of light in the life process.

Plants that are threatened by the devitalizing effects of climate, time of the year, poor soils, etc. form a lot of Vitamin C, and this is also true of our cowslip. The battle of cosmic enlivenment with sluggish protein processes that are overly exposed to earth forces becomes manifest in the formation of Vitamin C.

Cowslip root smells like anise and parsley leaves and it contains salicylic esters. Salicylic acid and its derivatives are mainly found in plants that come out of a damp and cool ground, but that want to dissolve into the light and air realm in a particularly intensive way with an active flowering process. In such plants the astral sphere that approaches the flowering process moves in powerfully from the airy region and transforms the vegetative impulse into a flowering one, that is, it works particularly strongly into the cool, watery sphere and it wrests this formation of flowers from it. One could mention willow, birch, wintergreen, pansy, pyrola, and meadow sweet here; these plants with many flowers all live in wet meadows, moor lands, woods, along rivers and seashores in cooler regions. Salicylic acid is soluble in water and it volatiles in steam. It inhibits the multiplication of yeast cells and other parasitic life and thereby inhibits fermentation. [33]

Remedies from cowslip flowers will work upon the metabolic system in such a way that it will assist the building up, nutritive and enlivening processes in the organism's "vernal region", and it will oppose and harmonize the hardening, paralyzing, "wintry" processes in the upper organization. Summer flowers and flowers in general work upon metabolic processes, vernal flowers work upon rhythmic processes, and winter flowers work upon those in the upper organization. The meeting of the blood with breathing and the enlivening permeation of the food that is becoming blood with the oxygen that brings in the forces of the etheric world is promoted. The building up and enlivening processes in the rhythmic system are stimulated and the heart and lungs are nourished better. Plants that intensively carry out the battle between levity light and gravity darkness in their organizations, as our cowslip so obviously does in its flowers, are very often ones that can heal heart ailments.

---

[33] See the discussion of willow species.

Its roots combine salicylic esters and a saponin content and they often help one to get rid of colds in the lungs, if the latter have taken in too many cold influences without elaborating them, have become too similar to sense organs, and have thereby been taken hold by the forces of the upper organization.

Anagallis arvensis – Scarlet Pimpernel

The time of the year has advanced again, the type no longer forms rosette plants, but lets the shoot stretch out as a stem. The tendency to creep along the ground is still there, but the rhythmic plant that is equipped with simple, little, oval leaves with pointed tips rises up a half a foot or more and puts out flat, purplish red (sometimes blue), little flowers on slender peduncles out of the leaf axils. Thus the rhythm of the leaves and the formation of the inflorescences are fused. The annual plant flowers from June to end of September; the flowers only open during clear, sunny weather, from about 9 a.m. to 3 p.m. This is the time of day when temperature, barometric pressure and other weather factors are more prominent.

A small, dry, spherical capsule proceeds from the flower as a fruit, which bends downwards towards the earth through a corresponding curvature of the peduncle.

Our plant loves fields, where it grows up in the shadow of damp grass blades and blooms after the hay is mowed. It also likes gardens, waste lands and soils that are bare after being cultivated, etc. If these places become covered with herbs and grass, our plant soon disappears.

The flowers contain anthocyanin dyes, and the sap contains an enzyme that digests protein, bitter substances and tannins. That is why the plant has a sharp, bitter taste.

A human being is "capable of getting sick" through the forces with which this soul and spirit prepares one's physical body to be the foundation of a consciousness processes. This is brought about through degradative and disintegration processes, especially in the nervous system. The healing effect of the upbuilding blood that is carried by iron must constantly oppose this. Iron is present in hemoglobin in an almost mineral (crystallizable) condition that is, however, entirely controlled by the I organization. With it the latter opposes the disintegration of protein

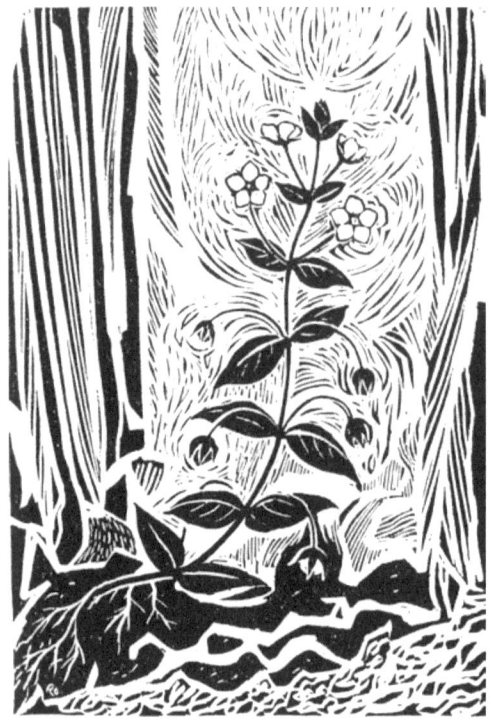

in nerves that is brought about through the astral body, controls it and keeps it within healthy limits.

If the astral body takes its degradative tendencies beyond the nerve region and, say, into the intestinal region, congestions and pains arise; a corresponding, balancing I activity has to be opposed to its hyper-activity. A substance like the iron in blood that tends to be on the mineral side must be put at its disposal for this purpose, but one that has a connection with the intestinal region. The alkali metals are such substances; if they are combined with sulfur processes they bear a force in them that inserts protein into the organism's life processes.[34]

Anagallis has such processes in it. It has a potassium process in its stems and a sulfur process in its flowers. They are pressed into each other in a perceptible way. Its peptonizing enzymes point to the degradation of proteins, and the saponins promote reaborption in the digestive region, as we mentioned before. Its bitter substances promote a healthy digestive process. The human digestive process has the same 9 to 3 o'clock rhythm that anagallis has in its flower process, although it falls out of it during "abdominal congestions". During this time the earth organism breathes forces out into the atmosphere that permit the atmospheric pressure to drop from its maximum at 9 a.m. to its minimum at 3 p.m. (daily, double atmospheric pressure wave). It goes into its "exhalation" phase. Man has

---

[34] We are following the text in chapter 7 of I. Wegman/R. Steiner's *Fundamentals of Therapy* here.

equivalent rhythms in the organs of his lower organization, especially in their etheric foundation. (The lower part of our etheric body is much more connected with the streams and rhythms of the earth's etheric body and of the etheric world than the upper, much more independent part is.) The organs in the lower organization oscillate in the same rhythms of exhalation and excretion from 9 a.m. to 3 p.m. that the earth's etheric body has; then comes the reabsorbing, inhalation phase that goes from 3 p.m. to about 3 or 4 a.m. If these rhythms occur too slowly (while the slower rhythms of the upper organization brought about by the way that the astral body in the nervous system works together with the etheric body, become displaced into the intestinal region or other parts of the lower organization), one gets congestions and hindrances to healthy rhythms.

Anagallis is an important remedy for such pathological conditions. It is probably no accident that this primrose that had fallen out of favor as a medicinal plant (a modern herbal) for the last two centuries, is the first to be mentioned by I. Wegman/R. Steiner in their *Fundamentals of Therapy*.

Lysimachia nummularia – Moneywort

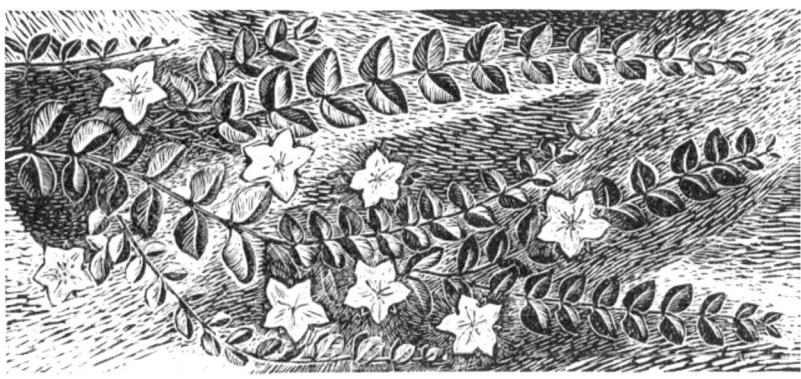

This friendly primrose flourishes in the early summer in damp, somewhat shady places; it likes wet ditches, damp lawns, watersides and meadows with short grasses. It unfolds its whole life flat on the ground. The reddish shoots drive out into the light from small roots; the quadrangular, winged stem process creeps over boggy ground and tightly holds little, rounded, golden green pairs of leaves. The internodes become longer and the leaves get bigger; the flower buds eventually grow out of the leaf axils, usually two at a node (see Roggenkamp's drawing), which open up into broad, golden yellow flowers with that characteristic primrose smell. The first leaves soon wither and the next ones turn brown, but new internodes keep on pushing out, until the activated flowering process stops the stem growth. The flowers and leaves like to turn towards the light. The flowers usually produce no fruits, the withering flowers turn towards the earth. However, now that the flowering process is over, the stems begin to grow again; the force that doesn't get turned into seeds goes into the branching growth of the ends of the shoots. Short internodes form and develop leaves and roots; the plant breaks up into many plants forming horizontal arcs or circles. A golden green wreath is woven on the ground and eventually it can cover it as a living layer of "skin". The leaves retain their simple, rounded form in all of these stages; one sees hardly any change in them where the flowers are. Thus it is clear that the vital pole of root and shoot is predominant over the flower pole and its astral impulses.

One can see the relation of our plants to light through the fact that its ashes are about 30% silica. Like all primroses, it also contains saponins, and we have often discussed their effect upon skin and blood. The silicic acid process that is always moving out peripherally into the sensory sphere directs the effects of the saponins and tannins that are in lysimachias into the skin. A Pfeifferian copper chloride crystal picture shows that our plant is a typical silica plant, with a central point and strong peripheral radiations; it is a "nerve-sense picture", like one gets from animal sensory and nerve organs. This material dynamics in moneywort enables one to understand why remedies made from it help one to control the blood process out to the skin's periphery and to place nutrition and shaping, or metabolic forces and formative forces in the right relation to each other. Our lysimachia has lush, yellow flowers and so what Rudolf Steiner once said about European cowslip and other flowers also applies to it. He said that such lush, yellow flowers promote the passage of the nutritional juice into the blood and also into the organs. In our case, this would mainly be into the skin organ, thanks to the silicic acid effect, especially if its effect is reinforced by another plant. Rudolf Steiner once indicated the use of such a preparation that was made from moneywort and bittersweet nightshade (Solanum dulcamara).

Cyclamen purpurascen [35] *– Sowbread*

The primrose being especially takes hold of the earthy element in the 30 cyclamens that grow in the eastern Mediterranean region, of which only C. purpurascens has moved up into the Alpine regions and slightly further north. This gives it a particular connection with permanence, darkness, gravity and inhibited growth, all of which it overcomes in primrose fashion.

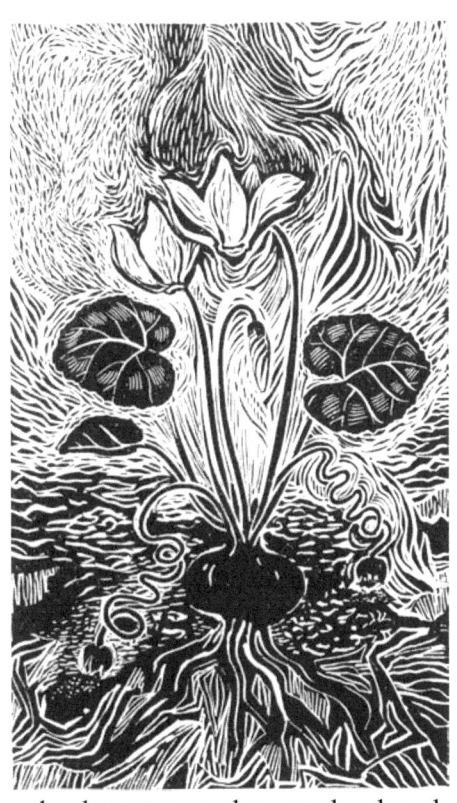

Its hypocotyl (the part between the root and the cotyledons) becomes a subterranean tuber. The first leaf develops slowly and the second small one comes quite a bit later, and then a few more leaves arrive. They are articulate and reminiscent of hearts and kidneys, slightly indented, on a long petiole, carmine red underneath, and a shiny, dark green above with silvery white stripes and spots that play gently over the blade in harmony with the leaf form, like spots of sunlight over a shady ground. Cyclamen looks for shade in bushes or woods and for the warm moisture that is best guaranteed by rocky, calcareous soils with humus.

The leaves always stay green, the shoot stays underground and sends up only leaves for the first few years, and then beautiful and fragrant, purple flowers. The buds of the latter rise freely from the ground on a spirally unrolling stem that gets about six inches high, and they nod down to the earth and stay in that position; however, the unfolding petals rise

---

[35] Cyclamen europaeum

upwards, giving rise to a rather unique flower form that is nevertheless quite primrosian, for it gives expression to its battle between levity and gravity. The bright purplish red shine that is already anticipated on the undersides of the leaves is the color with which darkness becomes resurrected in the light[36]. It arises if one looks through a prism at a dark strip on a white background, as soon as the prism works strongly enough so that it fuses the colored edges into a unity. It has a sweet and dry scent that is strong and delightful at the same time, evanescent and persistent, and it is not at all related to the wet moldy places it grows in. Thus the earthy plant is permeated by strong blossom power, and it has its full share of the airy, astral element. The fruit is a dry capsule, and it is drawn down by a spiral, curling movement that presses it into the ground; it pops open there and gives its seeds to the ants, who carry them off and stash them in clefts and fissures.

The entire plant, especially the tuber contains a lot of saponins and therefore it is toxic. Corresponding to the tuber formation, the healing effect is upon the head region, against goiter, migraines and similar headaches, and corresponding to its intensive flowering process, it heals the lower organization, aberrations in rhythms and menstrual congestions.

TYPICAL PHENOTYPES OF MEDICINAL PLANTS FOR THE LIVER, KIDNEY, LUNGS AND HEART

Earlier on we tried to arrive at the concept of extra corporeal "organs" of plants, terrestrial, cosmic force realms that steer plant life and that are just as important for this as our inner organs are for our bodily processes.

We will now try to approach the nature of medicinal plants for particular organs from a different side, and to press forwards to something typical from an overview of many such plants.

---

[36] See Goethe's *Theory of Color*.

Medicinal Plants for the Liver

Let us try to arrive at the characteristics of medicinal plants for the liver through concepts that arise when one looks at the liver organ and its activities. We should especially keep the following three things in mind.

1. The liver is the largest gland in our body and thereby it has a special place in our fluidic organism and in the formative forces or etheric body that organizes the latter. Fluids are assigned to the "chemical ether" that is one of the four kinds of formative forces; and in fact, the liver is a center for biochemical processes in the organism; Rudolf Steiner had good reasons for calling it the "chemist" among the organs.

2. The liver also has a special place in our warmth organization; it is the warmest organ in the body and its constant temperature of about 106°F (41°C) would be a very high fever in the rest of the organism.

3. The liver process continuously keeps a balance between its feverish activities. Condensation and dissolution, the formation and transformation of substances are continuously seething in the organic retort of this mysterious, powerful organ. One can see this particularly clearly in its dealings with carbohydrates that are condensed to glycogen or starch and then dissolved into sugar again and put back into the bloodstream.

We encounter these three properties in a unique way in the realm of inorganic existence in metallic tin[37]. Inner fluidity (malleability) and inner solidity and formative power (crystallinity) have been brought to a wonderful equilibrium in metallic tin. Tin retains its fluidic condition longer than any other warm metal over a range of 2068°C (m.p. 232°, b.p. 2300°). This is somewhat willful with respect to warmth. Once it has heated up to a certain point it defends itself against further heating by strengthening its form power; it becomes hard and brittle. It defends itself against too much cooling by an inner expansion and loosening and it becomes light and powdery.

If one sees that such properties are characteristic of the tin process, one can then call the liver process a tin process at an organic human level. One can see why tin is a basic remedy for the liver, with which one can oppose an overflowing vitality of an etheric organization that has become

---

[37] See the author's *The Secrets of Metals*, Anthroposophic Press

too strong, and also maintain an equilibrium between the physical and the etheric in general and between hardening and swelling.

This tin process can also be present in plants.[38] It will become manifest in particular relations of fluids to solids, in the characteristics of the play of forces between condensation and dissolution in the carbohydrate process in particular, and also in an obvious connection of plants with warmth processes. However, these are characteristics that one repeatedly finds in medicinal plants for the liver.

Plastic forms and swelling growths tell one about the activity of etheric forces in fluids; this is opposed by a strong formative power that can lead to peripheral hardening and a production of thorns. An independent, inner, fluidic plant is often secreted inside the outer, solid one, so that a plant with milky sap forms. Just think of plume poppies, fumitory celandine and other poppy like plants, of many compositae especially from the sub family of milky ray flowers like dandelion and chicory, and of artichoke, milk thistle and other "liver thistles".

A carbohydrate process that proceeds in a particular way is also characteristic of many medicinal plants for the liver. More soluble kinds of starch that one finds in most plants are formed in them, and they are closer to the kind of starch that is in liver. One finds inulin in most composites and galactans in the labiates that permeate this process with the warmth process that are peculiar to them. One finds inositol, a kind of a (ring) sugar, in other medicinal plants for the liver, and it is also present in livers and muscles. It is contained in grape leaves and in compositae.

The life processes of other groups of medicinal plants for the liver are connected with characteristic warmth effects; the ones that connect their carbohydrate processes with such life in warmth activities are particularly interesting. This is the case for grape vines and for certain members of the rose family. One should mention strawberry and grapes here that are the basis for the liver remedy that Rudolf Steiner recommended.

The connection between the carbohydrate and warmth processes stimulates the I organization to work into the liver activity in a proper way; for the I especially permeates the body's warmth processes.

---

[38] In that case it is present as a pure activity and not as a substance; one will not necessarily be able to detect the presence of any ponderable amounts of tin.

Another striking thing about many medicinal plants for the liver is that they produce a lot of bitter substances. Rudolf Steiner tells us that the latter "make the etheric body inclined to take the astral body into it". (See the indices in Volumes I and II under "bitter substances"). Bitter substances stimulate a liver organ that is living in the fluidic, etheric element too much to connect itself sufficiently with the activities of the astral body in degradative and excretory processes that lead to the secretion of bile and other things. (Rudolf Steiner once called bile an astral activity that has become physical.) The liver's "appetite" is increased by bitter substances; the organ becomes more interested in foods from the outer world, which is a condition for healthy digestion.

The beautiful and often showy flowering processes in plants that form bitter substances, point to the intensive intervention of astral realms into the physical and etheric bodies. Just think of gentians, bitter grounded citrullus colocynthis (bitter cucumber) and other cucurbits, the airily pinnatified worm woods, thistles and the quinine tree. However, these flowering processes are weak, and the astral element that produces them could not overpower the etheric, break through it, penetrate the physical, degrade and destroy protein, and generate alkaloidal poisons. The astral is taken in by the etheric body that is inclined towards this kind of thing and is completely worked through.

*

We will now give brief indications about the most important medicinal plants for the liver, arranged according to the following. A short description of the typical features of each family can give the reader an idea of its greater or lesser "proximity to the liver". For more details, see the chapter on the particular families.

I. Composites Compositae

The composite family contains a large number of liver remedies. This is due to its whole etheric configuration and to the peculiar way that the four kinds of ether interact in it. The characteristic thing that we found for the tin process becomes particularly manifest in this plant family: the equilibrium between fluidic and solid elements, plastically soft things and almost crystalline ones, and the resistance to excess heat and cold. There is a lot of milky sap formation, combined with the formation of thorns in thistles and in a few others. Inulin and other special kinds of starch are formed. We will give a few examples.

1. *Artichoke, Cynara Scolymus*: A plastically vital being that grows rampantly becomes congested, goes in to the form of a thistle, and wrests a magnificent flowering process out of the astral sphere as it fills itself with bitter compounds. The plant contains the starch inulin, like most composites, and inositol, a ring sugar; the sap also contains digestive enzymes. Artichoke preparations give a strong stimulation to building up processes via the liver, and they also promote bile flow.

2. *Blessed thistle, carduus benedictus*: This typical thistle with its congested growth, with flowerheads pressed deep into the plastic region of the leaves. Mucilages, tannins and bitter compounds combat liver congestions, jaundice and hemorrhoids. ; Rudolf Steiner indicated its use together with peony root as a new kind of remedy against edematous conditions.

3. *Dandelion, Taraxacum officinale*: What a wonderful interaction exists between flow and compression in this plant which is full of milky juice. One can easily discover the plastic, fluid element in this plant that is full of milky juice, also the strong formative power in the shape of the leaves, what a wonderful interaction between flow and compression. The plant's strong silica process opens it to the inraying cosmic forces of light, warmth and the effects of the superior planets, where Jupiter is predominant, as one can see from the flower's yellow color. Light and warmth work deeply into the life chemism in the milky juice that creates fats, waxes, inositol, inulin and many other substances.

Dandelion is used for liver conditioned edemas, jaundice, congestion in the portal vein and gallstone formations.

4. *Milk Thistle, silybum marianum*: One uses the slimy, bitter seeds from this thistle that cures the liver, and that has a mighty, congested, hemispherical bunch of leaves, out of which the long stemmed flower heads rise in order to combat hemorrhoids congestion in the portal vein region, and liver and bile blockages.

5. *Yarrow, Achillea millefolium*: On one hand, great vitality is wrested from an active flowering process; the shape that is imprinted on the solids, with tough stems and the thick ribs on the leaves that nevertheless allow the latter to be very fine and feathery; the tart juice, mild bitterness and gentle spiciness; shooting force in the herb and permanence in the umbrellas of flowers, all of these speak of how well the

opposing features in this fine plant are fit together into a harmonious unity. Rudolf Steiner said that the marvelous bringing together of potassium and sulfur processes in it was the important thing. It promotes the liver's activity that builds up the blood.

6. *Hemp agrimony, Eupatorium cannabinum*: The name Eupatorium refers to Mithridates Eupator, a King of Pontus who was a renowned concocter of herbal remedies. (*A Modern Herbal* p. 13; *Magic and Medicine of Plants*, p. 116). The name Hepatorium refers to the Greek word for liver – "hepar". This plant keeps a balance between solidity and fluidity in damp places along rivers and lakes; its shape becomes airy and divided at its top. Its bitter substances draw the astral sphere into the etheric realm. The plant is indicated for ascites and edematous conditions; the astral body that is induced to work in more intensively excretes the fluids that are becoming dead.

7. *Chicory, Cichorium intybus:* The life processes of this important medicinal plant for the liver plays back and forth like time between fluidic and solid, soft and hard, and alkaline and acidic (silicic acid). The plastic, milky juice is led over into tough stems. Its peculiar flowering process unfolds with morning sun, disappears with the afternoon sun and reappears the next morning as the flowers open again, in harmony with the cosmic 6 a.m. – 3 p.m. rhythms that are reflected in the liver's rhythms. (See Guenther Wachsmuth's *Earth and Man*.) According to an indication by Rudolf Steiner this bitter plant and the liver carry out their carbon processes in similar ways. (The root's high inulin content would seem to indicate this.) – Chicory—especially if it is fertilized with tin—supports the liver's action, increases the flow of bile and combats all inflammatory processes in the abdomen.

II. Mustards – Cruciferae

A rampantly growing and plastically swelling vegetation is taken hold of by sulfuric warmth and is permeated by sulfur here. Ripening heat forms a lot of fatty acid oil. That is why radishes and watercress are used to stimulate sluggish livers and to loosen congestions in the gall bladder region.

III. Lilies – Liliaceae

This plant family is characterized by sculpted, fluidic swelling, and by a carbohydrate process that leads to the formation of sugar and not of starch, which latter formation is a kind of a hardening of the process. Swelling congestion is followed by a vehement shooting into inflorescence. One could say that lilies are a watery inflammation that is accelerated by an intensive sulfur process. Water, warmth and carbohydrates in the liver tell us what this organ is all about.

1. *Aloe* is the mightiest of lilies and it gets impulses from Jupiter and Mars. This succulent plant lives in hot and dry landscapes with a formation of massive, swollen leaves that are filled with slimy juice and yet are hardened at the periphery; it is etherically congested for a long time until the tension is released by a fiery, blooming rocket. The formation of a lot of bitter substances prepares the etheric body that is closed off into itself to eventually take the astral into itself after all.

Aloe removes water, stimulates the liver, warms through the etheric, fluidic element and stimulates the flow of bile.

2. *Yucca filamentosa*: This lily also holds its plastic fluidic element down on the ground in an early battle with hardening tendencies, and it eventually uncoils almost explosively in its powerful inflorescence, whereby large amounts of sugar stream upwards. It takes in strong warmth effects in its subtropical home.

These processes enable it to do something for swelling of the liver, bile stoppage, jaundice and stone formations.

3. The common onion, *Allium cepa*, promotes the flow of bile.

IV. Labiates – Labiatae

The deeply intervening warmth processes that result in the formation of corresponding "warmth substances", essential oils in the herb, and fatty oils in the seeds are characteristic of the whole family. The flowering processes and scent formation are pressed into the region of the leaves and stem. Labiates also have an intensive process that forms sugar and starch that can be seen in the formation of much nectar (bees love dem plants), and in the deposition of galactans, an easily digestible kind of starch (in species of the stachys genus).

1. *Marjoram*: combats congestion in the portal vein and in the liver.
2. *Marrubium vulgare (white horehound)*: stimulates the liver and all its functions

3. *Peppermint*: enhances liver action and bile flow.
4. *Rosemary*: alleviates liver congestion, jaundice and diabetes.
5. *Cat Thyme*: fires up the liver process and promotes bile flow.

V. Poppies – Papaveraceae

These are swelling plants with plastic, roundish forms that are full of juice. Digestive enzymes that are useful in the human metabolism are found in the latter.

Overly strong astralization processes work into this rampant vitality to the point of poison formation and they congest the life functions and are pressed back again; unblocking of growth battles with congestion. Warmth processes in the ripening eventually overcome the poison process and imprint themselves on the seeds with the formation of fatty oils.

1. *Bloodroot – Sanguinaria canadensis* – stimulate action in the liver and gall bladder, and thereby relieves the upper organization from an excessive inflow of metabolic products that create migraines.

2. *Fumitory – fumaria officinalis – earth smoke*: helps in congestions of the liver, portal vein and bile.

3. *Celandine*: regulates the intervention of the astral body in the liver function, promotes the flow of bile, combats hardening tendencies and gets rid of astral cramp in this part of the body.

VI. Night Shades–Solanaceae

This plant type is characterized by an astrality that penetrates in an abnormal way, and it produces a lot of poison in vital saps that swell things up. Fruit formation fluctuates between smaller and bigger, dry and juicy berry forms (belladonna, tomato), dried out capsules (tobacco, henbane) and the dry, spicy capsule of jimson weed. The battle between swelling power and hardening addresses the liver organ; hardening tendencies are combatted and an astral element that works too strongly into the liver and gall bladder region and that becomes manifest in biliary colic and other cramps is liberated.

VII. Rose family – Rosaceae

What gives this family a connection with the liver is an interaction of carbohydrate and warmth processes, combined with a strong flowering process that points to the metabolic region right from the start. One should mention Fragaria vesca or strawberry, whose leaves and those of grapes are the basis for a remedy for the regulation and rhythmization of the whole liver process, according to an indication by Rudolf Steiner.

Agrimony, Agrimonia eupatoria, was used for the liver in ancient times and it continued to be an important liver remedy throughout the Middle Ages.

Rudolf Steiner once recommended a preparation of almond oil and essential oil from rose petals for cirrhosis of the liver.

VIII. Spurges – Euphorbiaceae

These are often plants with a congested, plastic, fluidic organization that produce a sharp tasting milk with strong warmth processes. They live their life in a strong tension between etheric and astral forces and between succulence and blossoming inflammation. One should mention herb mercury and the corresponding stillingia (Queen's Delight) in the tropics as remedies for liver ailments and skin disease that are connected with the liver.

MEDICINAL PLANTS FOR THE KIDNEYS

The kidneys (and adrenal glands) are metabolic organs that are mainly active in the fluidic organization and that are connected with the activities of the chemical ether or the biochemical activity of the etheric body. A large part of the kidneys' function involves the excretion of fluids and the replacement of most of what was excreted. However, they also have a more hidden but just as important connection with the airy organization and with the activities of the light ether in gases. The kidneys use seven times as much oxygen as the muscles that are connected with the skeleton, for instance. Malfunctions of the kidneys become manifest in respiratory disorders and in flatulence. Rudolf Steiner spoke of a very close connection of the kidneys to the whole air organization and to the human soul member that permeates it and lives in it, the astral body. For the latter, and therewith the air organization, is inserted in the metabolic system's building up activities by the kidney process.

The connection to the light ether is expressed through the function of the adrenal glands which manifests in the skin pigmentation.

The kidneys are sense organs, albeit subconscious ones, in addition to being metabolic organs. They must perceive the inner constitution of the blood stream that flows through them, in order to pick out what they are going to excrete. They also have deep connections with our sense organs for light, the eyes, some of which have been known to medicine for a long time, although we now know more about this through the discovery of the laws of metamorphosis in human organs (first from Goethe and then from the work of Rudolf Steiner).

These two functions that work together in the kidney process, the one in the metabolism that builds things up and the subconscious sensing activity, find a support in the dynamics of two substances, whose polar forces also are used in the biological processes of plants, animals and humans. The reader has encountered these two repeatedly in this book, sulfur and silicic acid. Without getting too redundant we should remember that sulfur stimulates the vitalization of the protein process and brings the latter to respiratory processes, whereas silicic acid strengthens formative forces, stimulates sensory functions and thereby promotes the permeation of things with light. Sulfur distributes the effects of silica over the whole organization and keeps them from accumulating too much around any one organ, which would isolate it from the body's other organs.

All of the characteristics of the kidney process that we just mentioned are reflected in the various medicinal plants for the kidneys in some way. If one tries to survey the large number of these plants, a common type arises before the mind's eye that deviates considerably from the liver plant type. Generally speaking, plants in the families that are related to the I and that have strong carbohydrate and warmth processes will often heal the liver, whereas many plants of strongly astralized families with their aeration and aromatization processes and protein formation processes that approach the animal nature can cure the kidneys. Of note here are legumes, carrots and madders (Leguminosae, Umbelliferae and Rubiaceae).

Another characteristic feature of medicinal plants for the kidneys is the way that their formative forces organization deals with liquids. They suck in a lot of water, but it is never stored up in succulent way; it is primarily exhaled into the air. The water that is assigned to etheric, formative forces is handed over to the air and the astral sphere. This type of plant tries to go beyond this and to incorporate airy things into itself by developing hollow spaces.

Many medicinal plants for the kidneys have an intensive silica process and some of them also have a strong sulfur process. We already indicated what this means for the kidney process. Plants of the Saxifrage family and a few other herbs add a balanced calcium process to the silica process so that they fit together quite well. Such plants have been used to combat gravel and stone formation in the kidneys for millennia.

We will place a detailed description of a prototype of medicinal plants for kidneys, field horsetail, at the beginning of our survey.

I. Field Horsetail – Equisetum arvense

A piece of earth history is projected into the present in equisetum, a memory of Nature of a plant in the far distant past that was still unable to produce flowers and that made the first, big step towards our green plants out of a more animal plant condition. It still has a more primal relation to minerals, water and light than the flowering plants do. Our ferns, horsetails and club mosses are the last remnants of a large number of plant forms that were created by a young and live earth in that part of its past that Rudolf Steiner described as the Lemurian epoch. In accordance with the basic biogenetic law, this childhood epoch repeated much older forms of existence in creation, especially those of the Old Moon, on which the only nature kingdoms below man were of a mineral-plant and a plant-animal nature. These old forms of life were repeated during the Lemurian epoch, although they were adapted to the new creative impulse that came in with typical, earthly conditions. A mineral kingdom was separated

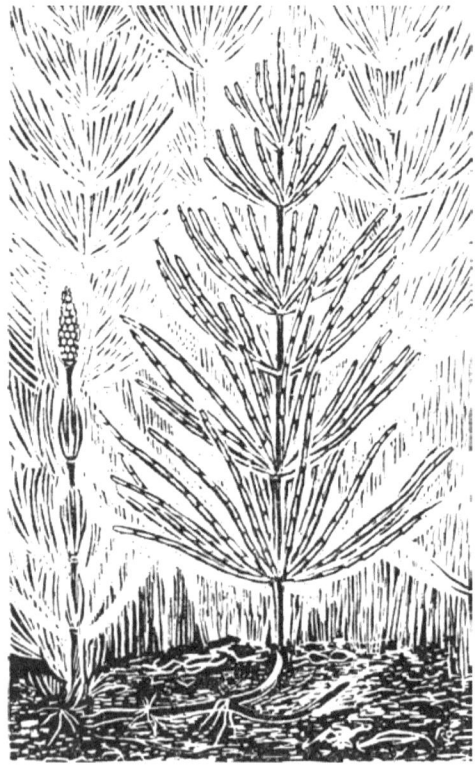

from these primal plants in a downward direction, the plant part of the animal was also expelled, and the inner connections of plants to minerals and animals were replaced by outer ones; roots and flowers arose.

There was no solid earth core during the Lemurian epoch; earth life unfolded in a vital atmosphere of very fine, fluidic, volatile albumin. Gigantic plant formations like algae swam in this atmosphere that had a lot of sulfur in it, and that was also permeated by silica processes that gave these plants cosmic formative forces. The mineral kingdom was then "devegetated" in a dramatic way, the siliceous materials were separated towards the earth's core, and rigidified into rocks; the sulfurous element was precipitated by metal processes radiating in from the cosmos and integrated into the rocks. The atmospheric albumin disintegrated; the fragments included oxygen, nitrogen, hydrogen and carbon, the present components of air.

Horsetail bears memories of those Lemurian processes in its life processes; with its crystalline, fine, siliceous shell and its fluids that are permeated by the sulfates of alkali metals, it is something like a living memorial to that time in which a tremendous purification and separation, a stripping off of a dead, old thing and a liberation for a new becoming occurred.

Field horsetail "flows" through orgilloceous, clayish–sandy soils with its multiply branched rhizome, as it sucks in much moisture and gives it over to the air. The pale, unbranched "flower" or club–shaped spore bearer that shoots out of it in the spring, looks parasitic and fungal like Indian pipe. After the spores have been dusted off it disappears and a grayish green, bushy stem springs up. Horsetail is all stem. The leafy element through which a plant opens itself to the airy region has disappeared almost entirely except for the serrations at the nodes. This airy region has been taken inside here. Whereas leaf buds are just barely indicated outwardly, air canals that are arranged around a central air space go through the entire plant and into all branches of its rhizome. Horsetail is permeated by much air and its pith consists of air. Thus watery and airy things have a particular relation to each other in it. This is also expressed by an intensive process that forms saponins that can mix watery and airy things into foam, and that also works physiologically wherever the fluidic and airy organizations intermingle. The saponin process is added to the strong silica process that would like to make our plant into a mineral formation almost entirely. The siliceous minerality seems to be kept within the plant's nature inwardly, but just barely; it becomes excreted at the periphery.

Horsetail's peculiar form also tells us something else. It looks like the extreme alkali plants that like to grow at the seashore, around salt mines and deposits at alkaline springs and on alkaline steppes. Look how similar it is to the glasswort Salicornia Europaea. However, there is an important difference between them. Real glassworts look watery and swollen, whereas horsetails with their alkali sulfates remain slender and rigid. As juicy as the latter are, they are controlled by formative forces. Salicornia looks edematous and horsetail looks like a Salicornia that has been cured of its edema.

Rudolf Steiner described the healing capacities of horsetail at various times, to the effect that this plant bears forces in the nature process that correspond to the building up forces in the kidney process. In the framework of comprehensive silica therapy he assigned it the role that arises from the interaction of vegetal silica processes and the sulfur processes that strive out of the life sphere into the mineral, salt condition. He gave many indications for the internal and external use of horsetail.

II. Borages – Boraginaceae

This family contains a lot of silicic acid and one of its members is gromwell, Lithospermum officinale, which has been used against kidney stones since the Middle Ages. It looks for damp, siliceous soils and sandy valleys with running water. Its hard nutlets contain a lot of silicic acid and calcium. The reader will find out more about what the connection between these two polar processes signifies in the chapter about stone breaks.

III. Carrot Family – Umbelliferae

It will not surprise the attentive reader that this plant family contains many medicinal plants that work upon the kidneys. These plants dissipate their watery contents in an aromatic way and radiate out the life force that is congested in their roots into the force tendencies of silica and in smaller and larger umbels. They connect with the airy region in many ways, as we can see from what was said about them in Volume I of Healing Plants.

1. Lovage, Levisticum Officinale, is a strong diuretic; it is used for edematous conditions and for stone ailments.

2. Creeping forget–me–not and other Eryngium species in which the type dares to go out into rocky places and begins to look something like a thistle, have been used for colds in the kidneys and bladder and for kidney colics and stones.

3. Parsley, Petroselinum hortense, has proven its value in stone ailments and urinary retention.

4. Celery, Apium graveolens, that grows along salty ocean shores, is engaged in a battle of airy light with salty dampness. It has been tried for ailments of the kidneys and bladder, stone formation and edema.

5. Water Pennywort, Hydrocotyle umbellata, lives in watery places with its airy umbels, and it is a strong diuretic.

IV. Legumes, Leguminosae

This plant family with its airy, sanguine nature intensively draws the astral realm towards it. Its particular way of forming protein, and its tendency to form inflammatory poisons, produces quite a large number of medicinal plants that work upon the kidneys, and we will pick out three characteristic ones.

1. Butcher's Broom, Sarothamnus scoporius: This plant holds back its leaf process in its green stems, and so its growth is something like that of horsetails. Like the latter, it contains a lot of silicic acid and it also exhales the water it has sucked up out into the air, and thereby intensively hands the water that is the vehicle of formative forces and their activities, over to the air that is the vehicle of the astral. The plant's many flowers also testify to the mighty activity of the astral realm in it. Broom has a diuretic effect, dissolves stones and relieves congestions in the fluidic organization.

2. Dyer's Broom, Genista tinctoria: This plant initially looks something like horsetail in its growth, and it is used for kidney and bladder ailments, cirrhosis of the kidney, the dissolution of gravel and stones and for edematous conditions that are connected with the kidney.

3. Rest–harrow, Ononis spinosa: This small, spiny, rigid plant with its many flowers looks watery and inflamed. It is used to combat urine retention, the storage of too much uric acid in gout, and stone formation.

V. Composites – Compositae

This large plant family contains strikingly few medicinal plants for the kidneys. We will only mention goldenrod, solidago virgaurea, that is used for nephro-sclerosis, uremic asthma, albuminuria, stone formation, and other things. It contains a lot of saponins.

VI. Madders–Rubiaceae

The madders are strongly astralized, just like legumes, and like the latter they take in nitrogen, the "astral's incarnation substance", directly out of the air. Their many species that attract ants, and the formation of substances that are related to uric acid also point to the astral realm. The rhythmic build up of its stems is somewhat similar to that in horsetail. Their species contain a lot of silica, and include a number of medicinal herbs for the kidneys.

1. Madder, Rubia Tinctorum, elaborates its high silicic acid content with potassium and calcium. In this plant the astral impulses in the flower region penetrate down into the mineral, root region that protects itself against this astralization through the formation of red dyes. When the latter are ingested as a medicine they make the patient's bones and urine red. The plant is used for kidney and bladder ailments and for kidney stones.

2. Coffee, Coffea Arabica, increases the astralization process of the Rubiaceae to the point where alkaloids are formed; caffeine is structurally related to uric acid.

3. Cleavers, Galium aparine, combines a large silicic acid content with the formation of saponins, that arise through the interaction of air and water processes. It has been used for urine retention, stone formation, edema and skin ailments that are conditioned by the kidneys.

4. Sweet woodruff, Asperula odorata, is indicated for gravel and stone formation.

VII. Mustard family – Cruciferae

The sulfur process that is so characteristic for the cruciferae is balanced with a polar salt process in some members of this family. For instance in shepherd's purse, capsella bursa pastoris, and in scurvy grass, Cochlearia officin. See Volume I for more details about these. In both plants the salt process presses upwards from the root into the formation of flowers. The first plant is salutary for bleeding of the kidneys and the formation of gravel and stones in the kidneys. The second one also combats the formation of kidney gravel, and it is used for urine retention.

VIII. Lily plants – Liliaceae

There are many medicinal plants for the kidneys in this family. They lead a slimy, watery congestion out into the intensive flowering process that shoots upwards and outwards, and in the process enclose air in hollow leaves or dissolve it in the airy region. Silica and sulfur processes are intertwined in many different ways.

1. Autumn crocus, Colchicum autumnale has been used to treat gout and the nephritis of scarlet fever.

2. Sea onion, Scilla (or Urginea) maritima: A delicate, but eventually quite long flower stalk is driven up out of a swollen, mighty onion. This plant is a strong diuretic and it is used for inflammations of the bladder and kidney.

3. Asparagus fern, Asparagus officinalis is again something like a horsetail that puts up a stem out of a unitary, yet much branched root system. It becomes very airy up above. Its silicic acid content is high. The plant has been used for gout, kidney and bladder ailments, and to combat stone formation.

4. Sarsaparilla, smilax medica, is a tropical plant that grows along rivers and puts up long vines into the air from a congested watery base in a mercurial, sulfuric way. It is used for inflammation of the kidney and bladder and for stones.

IX. Labiates – Labiatae

We know of only two medicinal plants in this "family of warmth plants" (see Volume I) that apply to the kidney. The kidney is the organ that inserts the astral body into the metabolic sphere. These plants balance the impulses of the astral sphere by emphasizing the cosmic, I, sun forces.

1. Orthosiphon stamineus, (Java tea) East Indian kidney tea keeps a balance between solidification and flowery inflammation in its outer appearance. It is used for chronic kidney inflammations, and to combat formation of gravel and stones.

2. Stingless Nettle, Lamium album (white dead nettle) is a labiate that has been toned down by a cool and damp element. It has been used on male geriatrics who retain urine.

X. Nightshades, Solanaceae

The only plant we'll bring in here is Chinese lantern, physalis alkekengi; because it has a formative gesture that can be seen in a number of medicinal plants. It has a red berry inside an inflated, airy calyx as in other formations with airy pockets, such as bladder campion and bladder wrack. This form is the expression of inner forces that reach over the fluids that are given to the plant and take hold of air. Like a number of such plants, Chinese lantern counteracts inflammations in the kidney and bladder region.

XI. Rose plants, Rosaceae

Rose hips contain a large amount of silicic acid. The swollen receptacles protect themselves against astralizing forces through their red color (Rudolf Steiner described the reddening of a rose blossom in this way). They enhance diuresis, if given as a tea, and combat the formation of stones.

MEDICINAL PLANTS FOR THE LUNGS

From a certain viewpoint the lungs are on organ that one needs to incarnate on earth. They are only acquired by breathing earth beings at a certain stage of development. As things pass over from gill to lung breathing, and the respiratory organs within the body, the limbs that enable one to move and to be active on terra firma are being projected outwards. The first breath is connected with a passage out of a fluidic life in the embryonic sphere into the world of heavy solids. The number of our daily breaths matches the average human life span in days: we breathe $18 \times 60 \times 24 = 25{,}920$ times a day, and this number of days is almost 71 years, or about an average lifetime. Rudolf Steiner often pointed to this significant connection. From the above we can understand why he related the constitution of one's lungs with the nature of the ground where one is living, and why he said that regions with particular rocks, such as the Vogel mountains (Hessen), are particularly healthy for the lungs.

Solids refer us to life ether and the breathing element is connected with light ether. These two kinds of formative forces are of the greatest importance for the life of the lungs.

Carbon is the earth substance that has the strongest connections with light and life ethers. It is connected with cosmic light processes through the plant's assimilation processes, and it is led into the solidification process of life ether that ends in the solid plant form. Carbon already shows its close connection with light and life ethers in the mineral realm, albeit only in a dead copy. In its diamond form it has the fieriest play of light and color and the greatest hardness among the earth elements. According to its constitution it should really be a volatile, transparent gas like oxygen and nitrogen, and many of its simplest compounds are just that, as one can see in any gas lamp. But by combining with itself as it does in diamonds, it condenses to the most solid thing of all.

There is nothing that compares with it as a chemical individual. The carbon compounds known to date far outnumber those of all other chemical elements combined. Its willingness to combine with other things, and then as a compound to combine with still more things seems to know no bounds. It is so inwardly plastic and capable of transformation, so ready to strip off old forms and to assume new ones at any time that it has become the basic substance in "organic" chemistry, and it also plays a significant role in organic chemistry.

"Chemical ether" is subject to the activity of "life ether" in it. Just as solids can maintain long term forms and can determine the shape of the fluids they hold as vessels, so life ether forms and determines the chemical ether that works in the flux of transformations of substances. That is why Rudolf Steiner also called this most mysterious kind of formative force "meaning ether", because it imprints the meaning, or the spiritually real principle of a life form into the chemical ether's chemism. Chemism is like a harmony or a composition of sounds (it is not for nothing that chemical ether is also called sound ether); however, life ether is superordinate to the sound medley, it gathers the many sounds and chords together into a motif, it is the musical movement.

This spiritual form that gives a meaning to things can become incorporated on earth, because carbon exists, with its close connection to meaning or life ether. Thus like its counter process, the plant's assimilation process, the lung process has the deepest connections with carbon, light and life ether.

After what was said above we would expect medicinal plants for the lungs to have a special way of dealing with light and life ethers and with the carbon process. The connection of some of these plants with light processes comes from the silicic acid they contain. One often notices the development of a lot of leaves and nodes in continuous rhythmic succession, so that there is little change in form from one end to the other. This indicates the existence of a mercurial principle in these plants that is sometimes reinforced by traces of metals and thereby a mineral, mercurial element. We can see a special way of dealing with carbon carbohydrates in the mucilage formation of some medicinal plants for the lungs. Plant mucilages are glucides or substances that are related to cellulose, although they don't lend themselves to solidification and hardening in the formation of wood. They hang on to water tenaciously and remain soft and plastic. Plants that form a lot of mucilage control their carbon or liquefaction process, and so they often are good fiber plants. This results in a special connection with life ether and the carbon process.

Man's lung organ has to maintain an equilibrium between the formative principles in the upper, sensory nervous organization and the dissolving principles in the lower, metabolic organization, and cannot give in to either hardening or softening impulses. Typical medicinal plants for the lungs keep a balance between formative, light and silica processes, and dissolving mucilage processes, etc.

For instance, just look at the somewhat strange labiate, sage–leaved germander, Teucrium scorodonia, that Rudolf Steiner was probably the first one in the 20th century to recommend as an important medicinal plant for the lungs. One can see it growing rampantly in the colored sandstone heights of the Black Forest, a region that has a good effect on lung patients. We can see that it is one of the main plants in those forests and a special harmony between the landscape and "its" plants is disclosed. Iron and silica processes are the basic forces that become manifest in the red sandy rock, both of which are light bringing elements in their own way. Because of the mountain landscapes they are surrendered to cosmic light processes. To an especially large extent the solid earth lights itself up into the atmosphere and towers into the light ether zone in an intensified way. Thus life and light ethers interact in a particular way.

The woods germander grows to its full strength on the edges of these elevated woods, in clearings and on wet, rocky places. It shoots up, narrow and tall, like a nettle; it towers up, node on node, leaf after leaf, and thereby shows that it likes to develop the rhythmic middle of the stem and leaf element. It responds to the iron in the ground in the same way that stinging nettle does. However, its large content of silicic acid helps to establish a special connection with light. For teucrium flees the full effect of the sun; it grows in fairly shady places, and it loves dim light (which is much better than bright sun light for lung patients). Our plant would have to shoot up as a pale weakling in such a place, if it didn't heal itself with silica and iron. The inflorescence lifts itself up as a pale, yellowish white spike, and it turns its individual flowers out of their unspecialized positions in the direction of the greatest light that is present in the twilight woods. However, the strong almost dark, nettle green of the leaves, that arose through light and out of the light with the help of iron tells us of a force that can even get light out of twilight.

Sage germander smells dully resinous and almost like sweat; the fiery aromatization process of normal, typical labiates (lavender, rosemary, thyme, etc.) is dampened by the woods' humus and the shady, damp nature of its growing place. The whole plant is also permeated by bitter substances. It stimulates lung patients' "organ appetite", which we mentioned in the introduction to this section on medicinal plants for organs. This plant also has a healing effect on the abnormal production of sweat in tuberculous patients through the special way in which warmth processes take hold of the dark and damp element in it and are dampened there.

Silica plants in which the silicic acid process is connected with a strongly emphasized rhythmic leaf and stem growth have been known as a source of drugs for lung ailments for a long time. For instance a popular mixture of teas consists of the dried herbs of horsetail, knotweed (polygonum aviculare) and common hemp nettle, all three of which grow in the way just described. Life ether and the condensed carbon process expresses itself in the contracted, solidified and lignified stem organ that lets new life germinate from each node.

Rudolf Steiner recommended a previously unused mixture of teas to promote better nutrition of the lung organs. This was a mixture of dried dark yellow flowers of plants that primarily live in flower formation, St. John's Wort, European cowslip and bird's foot trefoil. Flowers in general fire up the metabolism. The dyes in the yellow flowers mentioned are carotenes. We have often mentioned the latter in these volumes of *Healing Plants*. (See the indices.) They have a particular connection with light metabolism, the activity of light ether, and also with silicic acid's spheres of activity. They capture light and silicic acid processes in carbon substances, as it were. They transfer light energy to the green chlorophyll in leaves; for they are grouped around the chlorophyll process in the green leaf, although their color is blotted out by the green chlorophyll. However, in the yellow flowers mentioned these carotenes emerge from the greenness and stand by themselves. When used as remedies such flowers will give the metabolism an impulse towards rhythmic, light elements. (See what was said about European cowslip and St. John's Wort above). Carotene is converted into vitamin A in the human organism, that has to do with the enlivening of the whole ectoderm and the sphere of the sense organs that proceeds from it. We find the highest concentrations of this vitamin in our visual purple.

Another silica drug is lungwort, *Pulmonaria officinalis*, that blooms in the still leafless woods in early spring. This plant belongs to the borage family that combines silicic acid and mucilage forming processes. Here we come to another important feature in medicinal plants for the lungs. They often form plant mucilages that have long been valued for the expectorant effect that liberates lungs that are filled with mucus. Other plants we could mention here are marshmallow, elecampane, Iceland moss and butterbur. We already mentioned that plant mucilage is a kind of "liquid wood" or cellulose, and that we are dealing with a carbon process that avoids hardening.

Thus the reader has gotten used to seeing the lung and carbon processes in a certain connection. He will now be able to understand another indication by Rudolf Steiner, that a healthy lung process must generate a certain amount of mucous for other things besides the lung organ. For if this production of mucous is too little the head will tend to get certain diseases. (However, we can't go into this any further.) Iron silicate can help to cure things here. However if men must live in a climate with damp and cold air, the lung produces too much mucous. The leaves of certain kinds of cabbage can be used as remedies. Here the carbon process that always presses towards the bearing of shapes and structures wrestles with the dissolving, inflammatory sulfur process that always drives etherically enlivened things towards a permeation by air. These kinds of cabbage like a damp, cool climate, and they contain a lot of iron.

We can speak about coltsfoot, butterbur and wild sunflower (elecampane) in a similar way. A mighty leaf formation that is connected with a powerful subterranean or superterranean stem in rhythmic succession always stands out in such plants.

Thus a penetrating look reveals plant processes as counter images to human processes that form organs. On the background of larger connections we begin to understand the at first puzzling result of supersensible investigation that carbon is the external lungs for plants, and that the formative forces of the human lung organ are something like the highest organic manifestations of carbon. A type for medicinal plants for the lungs becomes visible and places itself at the side of typical plants for the liver and kidneys. Of course we are dealing with healing effects that assist the lungs' formative and building up forces, etc. However, some lung diseases result from disrupted functions and from more widespread diseases of the whole organism, rather than from deficient upbuilding. Bronchial asthma, emphysema and lung cancer would have to be treated by other kinds of medicinal plants.

Medicinal Plants for the Heart

A close look at many curative plants for the heart enables us to see a special type of plant that rhythmically weaves and lives in a kind of struggle between levity and gravity, and cosmic and terrestrial elements. We find a strong formative force life and a mightily onrushing astral region and the diastolic impulse of light and warmth ethers and the systolic tendencies of chemical and life ethers. The following description of major plants for the heart tries to explain this and to interpret their gestures.

Red Foxglove, *Digitalis purpurea*, condenses its entire growth into the formation of a large rosette of leaves on the ground in the first year, and as a counter thrust it shoots into a hyperactive flowering process the following year, that pulls the leaves up with it. The flower buds arranged in an upright position on all sides of the mighty spike of the central stem, open on the side where there is the most light. The deeply indented, bulging bells immediately sink down below the horizontal plane and eventually fall off as if they had been cut with a knife. Thereupon the ripening fruit capsule stands straight up and releases its tiny and very light seeds.

Key of Heaven, *Primula veris*, that especially belongs to the rhythmic spring time and to the Easter sun is really an image of the annual meeting of cosmic and earth forces. The short and strong rootstock that hangs on to its rosette of leaves belongs to the latter, whereas the long spikes of flower buds that are borne up lightly after winter's end belong to the former. Their rays turn towards the strongest light and nod down at the same time. Each flower arrives at its equilibrium position between levity and gravity as it opens, bows down and withers, and the fruit capsule lifts itself up again, strongly and almost stiffly.

The vernal, sunny, golden yellow flower contains carotene, the light substance. The plant's high saponin content is an expression of the dynamics with which the formative forces of the watery and airy elements mingle strongly whereby the March wind almost blows into its stream of sap. The flowers' delicate lemon scent breathes out its lightness and brightness, whereas the dull and sweetish methyl salicylate scent of its roots tells us of a battle with winter's cold and dampness in its gravity region.

Queen of the Night, *Cereus grandiflorus* is a cactus and a powerful heart remedy. It laboriously works the fleshy and long green jointed stems up along the limestone cliffs of islands in the Caribbean, constantly looking for holds with its crompons. The massive flower buds swell out mightily towards the sides, the long trumpets open for one night only, lifted slightly above the horizontal, but then they sink and wither. What a contrast between the rampant green growth that flows along steadily through the power of the hot daylight and the blazing up of the fleeting blooming action at night. The sun's power and the force of gravity fight a special battle in this plant, and so do the etheric, vegetative principle and the astral principle that works so strongly and violently into the flowering process.

The human head organization becomes strongly shaped in the dynamic tension between the physical and etheric elements. The sclerotizing, mineralizing element becomes prominent, the life forces are partly withdrawn from the physical body, and the sense organs become almost like physical apparati. However, the human mind thinks with these etheric formative forces that have become liberated in the earthly body.

The rhythmic system equilibrates the impulse of the etheric and astral bodies as they weave back and forth. It provides the bodily foundation for the feeling of the soul. Heart plants bear the motif of a strong tension between the etheric and astral in them, in addition to the light and heavy motif. One can see this particularly clearly in Queen of the Night.

Lily of the Valley, *Convallaria majalis*, is a plant where levity and gravity battle for a balance sometimes in slightly shady places under beeches, and the course of its life is also shaped by a strong tension between etheric and astral forces. For years only two leaves rise up out of a rhizome that continues to grow, until finally a leafless, narrow flower stem shoots up. Its end is surrounded by spirally arranged and upright flower buds. But then it obligingly bows down. The opening flowers all turn in one direction, towards the greatest brightness, which could even be north if the trees block off other light. The chalky white bells turn downwards and eventually all of them hang down under the force of gravity.

Strophanthus hispidus is a tropical plant for heart ailments and it has all of the characteristic features with which we've become acquainted. With its large, thick leaves it works its way upwards in the jungle as a luxuriant, herbaceous plant. It develops large flower buds that look like twisted candles on the last pairs of leaves on each shoot. Their long tips at the ends of flower petals that are wrapped spirally into pointed cones, directed vertically upwards, seemingly mocking gravity; when they open the long strings hang down and decorate the chalice in a strange way. Its seeds are light as a feather, with tails consisting of long, silky hairs.

*

Like the heart organ itself, plants that heal it are to a great extent under the influence of polar formative forces to a particularly large extent. They are molded in a special way by the systolic, contracting power of chemical and life ethers and the drastic, expanding power of light and warmth ethers. It is clear that they go through the rhythms of congestion and release from tension. Stimulation and dampening of life, vitalization and astralization, pulse through these plants in a particularly strong way. Terrestrial and solar forces battle each other and become harmonized in them. The hydrogen process becomes manifest in all of these essential characteristics. Compare this description of the type with what was said in the preceding chapter about the hydrogen process in connection with the heart's action. (The plant pictures that were outlined in the present summary are described in more detail in various parts of these two volumes of *Healing Plants*, see the indices. One also finds other heart plants like *Adonis vernalis* and *Crataegus Oxyacantha* there, which would have made the present section too long.)

By way of conclusion we will make a few comments about the so-called cardioglycosides or substances with very similar structures that people have found in many medicinal plants that work upon the heart. Chemists call these substances steroids because they have a complicated steroid ring consisting of carbon and hydrogen units as their nucleus. To the great surprise of scientists, they have found similar structures in cholesterol, bile acids, vitamin D, sexual hormones and in the very carcinogenic benzopyrenes in coal tar.

The steroid ring could theoretically be derived from oleic acid through condensation processes, and for plant life this points to the hydrogen process and warmth ether or to processes that finally culminate in the formation of fats and the development of seeds. From here one's gaze falls upon cholesterol, bile acids and the digestion of fats.

On the other hand, the solidification, calcification and bone forming processes that vitamin D initiates so energetically point to life ether and its condensation tendencies. One should also mention here the gallstone formations in which cholesterol is involved. The two poles of warmth and life ether between which the hydrogen process oscillates become manifest. They show up in a distorted way in the carcinoma process; one of the many ways to look upon the formation of tumors and metastasis is to regard them as pathologically distorted images of tendencies towards systolic concentration and diastolic scattering.

The reader will find more details about this interesting chapter on vital chemistry in the section on the snapdragon family (Scrophulariacea), where foxglove is discussed.

INDEX OF ILLUSTRATIONS

(To find the picture for a particular plant see the general index, where the page number is followed by an asterisk.)

Amanita caesareae	Royal agaric	12
Lobaria pulmonaria	Tree lungwort	16
Pteridium esculentum	Bracken	17
Aspidium felix–mas	Male fern	21
Pinus montana	Dwarf Pine	30
Larix decidua	European larch	32
Juniperus communis	Common juniper	35
Juniperus sabina	Spreading juniper	36
Hypericum perforatum	St. John's Wort	39
Saxifraga granulata	Meadow saxifrage	44
Chrysoplenium alternifolium	Golden saxifrage	45
Bryophyllum calycinum (or pinnatum)	Sprouting leaf plant	50
Sedum acre	Wall pepper	51
Dendrosicyos socotrana	Cucurbit tree	55
Byronic alba	European white bryony	58
Crocus sativus	Saffron crocus	61
Iris germanica	German Iris	63
Iris germanica	German Iris with flower	64
Oryza sativa	Rice	71
Saccharum officinarum	Sugar Cane	73
Hordeum sativum	Barley	77
Avena sativa	Oats	79
Agropyron repens	Couch grass	80
Arum maculatum	Lords and Ladies	85
Acorus calamus	Sweet flag	88
Quercus robur	English oak	95
Salix alba	White willow	101
Betula pendula	White birch	105
Citrus limonum	Lemon tree	109
Ruta graveolens	Rue	113

Dictamnus albus	Burning Bush	115
Saponaria officinalis	Bouncing Bet (soapwort)	117
Sambucus nigra	Elderberry	128
Hippophae Rhamnoides	Sea buckthorn	131
Copper chloride crystallization pictures of animal organs and medicinal plants		162
Eucalyptus globulus	Fever tree	165
Eugenia caryophyllata	Clove tree	167
Geranium robertianum	Herb Robert	169
Oxalis acetosella	Wood sorrel	173
Malva silvestris, var. mauritanica	Tree mallow	180
Digitalis purpurea	Foxglove	185
Verbascum thapsiforme	Mullein	192
Veronica officinalis	Speedwell	194
Gratiola officinalis	Hedge Lyssop	196
Scrophularia nodoso	Figwart	197
Convolvulus sepium	Bind weed	199
Olea europaea	Olive tree	203
Apocynum Cannabinum	Hemp dogbane	212
Nerium oleander	Oleander	213
Strophanthus gratus		214
Rauwolfia serpentina		215
Ledum palustre	Wild rosemary	219
Arctostaphylos Uva–ursi	Bearberry	221
Vaccinium Vitis-idaea	Cowberry (Mountain Cowberry)	223
Primula veris	Key of Heaven (Cowslip)	228
Anagallis arvensis	Scarlet Pimpernel	232
Lysimachia nummularia	Moneywort	233
Cyclamen purpurascens	Sowbread	235
Equisetum arvense	Field Horsetail	246

Index

A

Achillea millefolium 240
Achlamydeae.............................. 89
Acorus calamus 87, 89
Adonis 186
Adonis vernalis 259
Agaric....................................... 11
Agaricus comp./Phosphorus.......... 24
Agathosma 109
Agropyron repens........................ 80
Albuminuria 250
Alcohol............................. 122, 123
Algae 8, 14
Alkaloids 210
Allium cepa 242
Aloe... 242
Alpine roses 218
Amanita caesarea 13
Amentiflorae 89, 90, 91
Anagallis arvensis 231
Angelica 114
Anthocyanin dyes....................... 231
Antimony 78
Antipyretics.............................. 202
Apium graveolens 249
Apocynaceae 209
Apocynum cannabinum 211
Araceae 82
Araine....................................... 86
Arbor Vitae 33
Arbutin 219, 222, 223
Archetypal plant.......................... 50
Archichlamydeae 89
Arctostaphylos Uva ursi 221
Arsenic...................................... 40
Arsenic and astral body................ 41
Arsenic process 42
Arsenification............................. 42
Artichoke 240
Arum maculatum................ 82, 84, 86
Ascorbic acid 110, 135
Asparagus officinalis................... 251
Asperula odorata 250
Asthenia 16
Asthma 93, 250
Astral body... 93, 94, 103, 188, 243, 251

Aucubine 192
Aurantoidea 109
Averrhoa.................................. 174

B

Baby's breath 116
Balsamic resins........................... 30
Bamboo 82
Barley 77, 78, 79
Barosma betulinum 115
Bearberry................................. 221
Beech....................................... 91
Belladonna 114
Benzoic acid............................. 223
Betula pendula.......................... 104
Betulaceae 91
Betuline 105
Bilberry................................... 222
Bile acids................................. 188
Bindweeds................................ 198
Biophytum................................ 174
Biophytum sensitivum................. 174
Birch........................... 90, 91, 106
Bird's foot trefoil....................... 255
Bitter resins 56
Bitter root................................ 116
Bitter substances.40, 55, 65, 93, 111, 112, 194, 231, 232, 239
Bittersweet nightshade 234
Bladder ailments........................ 222
Blessed thistle........................... 240
Bloodroot 243
Blue Gum Tree.......................... 164
Boeletus mushroom..................... 11
Bombaceae 178
Boraginaceae 248
Boron...................................... 126
Boronioceas............................. 109
Bouncing Bet............................ 116
Bracken 87
Brain flu 13
Brazil cherry............................. 163
Bread 69, 71, 76, 143
Bryonia alba.............................. 57
Bryophyllum 47, 49
Bryophyllum calycinum 50
Buchu 115, 116

263

Buckwheat 90
Bufotoxin 186
Burns 42, 52
Butcher's Broom 249

C

Calamus root 84, 88
Calcium 78, 96, 97, 111, 112, 187, 189, 248, 250
Calcium carbonate 97
Calcium process 96, 97
Calla lily 84
Campions 116, 118
Caprifoliaceae 126, 127
Carbon 157
Cardioglycosides 212, 260
Carduus benedictus 190, 240
Carotene 111, 134, 229, 255
Carrot Family 248
Caryophyllaceae 68, 116, 118
Cat Thyme 243
Catch fly 118
Catkin bearers 89
Celastrales 90
Celery 249
Centrospermae 90
Cereus grandiflorus 258
Chemical and light ethers 27
Chemical ether 15, 59, 155
Chemical ether 253
Chickweeds 116
Chicory 241
Cholesterol 188
Chronic kidney inflammations 251
Chrysosplenium 45
Cichorium intybus 241
Cinnamon tree 163
Cissus 120
Citric acid 110, 112, 135, 175
Citrus limonum 109
Cleavers 250
Clove pink 90, 116
Clove Tree 167
Coat flower 116
Cockscomb 116
Coffea Arabica 250
Colchicum autumnale 61, 251
Colds 59, 76
Colics 88, 196
Colocasia esculenta 84

Combretaceae Combretums 91
Common hemp nettle 255
Compositae 90, 239, 249
Composites 249
Coniferae 25
Conifers 36
Constipation 22
Conthorellus ciborius 13
Convallaria majalis 259
Convolvulaceae 198
Corn 78
Corncockle 116, 118
Corylus Avellana 98
Couch Grass 80
Cowberry 222
Cramps 23, 114
Crane bills 168
Crassulaceae 47
Crataegus Oxyacantha 259
Crimson rambler 180
Crocus Sativus 61
Cruciferae 130, 241, 250
Cucurbitaceae 52
Cusparoideas 109
Cyclamen 198, 225
Cyclamen europaeum 62
Cyclamen purpurascen 235
Cynara Scolymus 240
Cypressaceae 33

D

Dandelion 240
Darnel 82
Dasheen 84
Desmodium gyrans 174
Diabetes treatment 32
Diaphoretic 103
Diarrhea 103, 196
Dictamnus albus 114
Digestive process 22
Digestive weakness 34
Digitalis purpurea 184, 257
Diosma 109
Diuretic 130, 249, 251
Dizziness 59
Dogbane Family 209
Dwarf Juniper 34
Dyer's Broom 249

E

Edelweiss 90
Edema 250
Edematous conditions 65, 66
Elderberry 126, 127, 129
Elderberry pith 130
Elephant's ear................................84
Entomophthorales 12
Epilepsy 87, 114
Equisetum arvense 246
Ericaceae......................................216
Essential oils .. 22, 27, 31, 33, 34, 65, 103, 107, 114, 129, 163, 169, 206, 242
Etheric body 155
Ethers 154
Eucalyptus....................................163
Eucalyptus globulus 164
Eucalyptus occidentalis...............164
Eugenia caryophyllata.........163, 167
Eupatorium cannabinum 241
Euphorbiaceae.............................244
Euphrasia officinalis 190
European cowslip........................255
European Cowslip 228
Evergreens.....................................25
Eyebright.............................. 184, 190

F

Fagaceae..91
Fagora 109
Feathered pink.............................116
Ferns 16
Feverish colds 103
Field Horsetail.............................246
Fig marigolds 171
Figwort.................................184, 197
Filicinae...16
Flavones 198
Fly agaric 11
Forgetfulness.................................59
Formic acid 176
Four o'clock 116
Foxglove 183, 184
Fraxinella 114
Fumaria officinalis 243
Fumitory......................................243
Fungi 10, 14, 18, 24, 81, 84, 122

G

Galium aparine 250
Garden loosestrife 225
Gencydo 112
Genista tinctoria 249
Geraniaceae.................................168
Geranium roberticum 170
Gerson diet..................................106
Gladiola...61
Glasswort 248
Glycerin.......................................207
Glycosides....................56, 198, 210
Goldenrod....................................249
Gourds...52
Gout....................... 221, 249, 251
Gramineae 66, 68, 81
Grape Family...............................119
Grapes 90
Grasses 66
Gratiola officinalis 195
Guttiferae 37
Gymnosperms 89

H

Hay fever.......................................76
Hay flowers 77
Hazelnut 98
Headaches 59
Heart..160
Heartburn 22
Heather Family............................216
Hedge Hyssop 184, 195
Hemp agrimony...........................241
Hemp Dogbane............................211
Herb Robert.................................170
Hernandiaceae...............................91
Herniary......................................116
Hippophae Rhamnoides 130
Honeysuckle........................126, 127
Horsetail...... 247, 248, 250, 251, 255
Huckleberry.................................222
Hydrocotyle umbellata 249
Hydrogen.....................................158
Hyoscyamus 114
Hypericine.............................40, 42
Hypericum perforatum 38
Hysteria 51

I

Inner light....................................157

265

Inositol 125
Iridaceae 60
Iris Germanica..............................62
Issima..127
I-strengthening effect 32

J
Jambolam plum 163
Jasmine..202
Juglandoceae..................................91
Juglans regia............................92, 93
Juniperus communis......................34

K
Kalmia latifolia 220
Kidney colics 249
Kidney gravel...............................250
Kidney stones................................47
Kidneys...157

L
Labiatae................................242, 251
Lack of appetite.............................88
Lacmellia edulis 210
Lamium album 251
Latherwort....................................118
Ledol 219
Ledum palustre............................219
Legumes.......................................249
Lemon Tree..................................109
Leontopodium alpinum 90
Levisticum Officinale..................248
Lichens...14
Life ether...............................15, 253
Light and warmth ethers...............27
Light ether.....................................15
Lilac 201
Liliaceae................................242, 251
Lily of the Valley 186, 259
Limestone and light processes.......43
Linnaea borealis 127
Liver..155
Lolium temulentum......................81
Lonicera 127
Lords and Ladies...........................84
Lovage 248
Lung..158
Lychnis viscaria 118, 119
Lysimachia nummularia......225, 233

M
Madder 126
Madders..250
male genital tract 221
Malic acid............................112, 135
Mallows..178
Malvaceae 178
Marjoram...............................97, 242
Marrubium vulgare.....................242
Marsh Rosemary 219
Marshmallow root 181
Meadowsweet..............................102
Meaning ether................................15
Merulius lacrimans.......................13
Metachlamydeae 89
Milk Thistle.................................240
Millet..71
Mimosa pudica 174
Moneywort....................................225
Monocotyledons............................89
Mountain Cranberry 222
Mountain Laurel..........................220
Mucilage.........................33, 60, 178
Mullein.................................182, 192
Mustard family 250
Mustards.......................................241
Mycelia 11
Mycetophyta..................................11
Myritaceae......................................91
Myrtaceae, Myrtles......................163

N
Nailwort 116
Nephro-sclerosis..........................250
Neurasthenia..................................51
Nightshades.........................243, 252
Nitrogen 155

O
Oak bark..97
Oats...79
Oil formation...............................203
Old Moon.....................................246
Oleaceae.......................................200
Oleander...............................186, 212
Olive Family 200
Ononis spinosa 249
Onopordon 190
Osteomalacia 13
Osteoporosis............................13, 23

Ouabain 210
Ovoid fruit trees 91
Oxalic Acid Process 170
Oxalidaceae..................................170
Oxalis acetosella 176
Oxalis hedysaroides 174
Oxygen..156

P
Paeonia officinalis........................190
Pansies 102
Papa Gontier.................................180
Papaveraceae................................243
Parasites 12
Parsley...249
Pearl weeds 116
Pearlwort.......................................116
Pelargonium zonale.....................168
Pepper...90
Peppermint 243
Petroselinum hortense 249
Phycophyta.......................................8
Pinaceae 30
Pine family 30
Pinks 116
Pipe tree 129
Piperoles...90
Pitch Pink 118
Plant acids 125
Polygonales....................................90
Poppies 243
Primula..190
Primula veris 228, 257
Primulaceae.........................118, 224
Primulas 102
Proranales.......................................89
Psolliota compestris 13
Psoriasis..33
Pulmonaria officinalis 256
Purslane..116

Q
Queen of the Night......................258
Quercus robur................................94

R
Ranales..89
Rauwolfia.....................................210
Rauwolfia serpentina...................215
Red Foxglove 257

Red Oak 94
Rest–harrow 249
Rheumatic complaints 59
Rheumatism 221
Rhododendron ferrugineum 220
Rice 77
Rickets......................................56, 88
Rockfoil....................................43, 47
Rosaceae...............................243, 252
Rose Bay 212
Rose family 243
Rosemary 243
Rubiaceae 126, 250
Rue..................... 107, 113, 114, 115
Rupture wort 118
Ruta graveolens...........................113
Rutaceae 107, 114, 115
Rutin..52, 114
Rye..71
Rye grass 81

S
Saffron Crocus 61
Salicaceae.....................................100
Salicoceae......................................91
Salicornia Europaea....................248
Salicylic Acids 224
Sambucus ebulus.........................126
Sambucus nigra 126, 127, 129
Sambucus racemosa 126
Saponins 79, 117, 198, 224, 226, 250
Saprophytes 12
Sarcocaulon 168
Sarothamnus scoparius...............249
Sarsaparilla 251
Saxifragaceae 43
Scarlet fever 10
Scarlet Pimpernel 231
Scilla 251
Sclerosis...78
Scrophularia nodosa 197
Scrophulariaceae 182, 195
Sea buckthorn......................132, 133
Sea Buckthorn..............................130
Sea onion......................................251
Sedum acre 51
Sedums 176
Shepherds purse 97
Silica 73
Silica Processes 43, 66

Silicates 74
Silicic acid 73, 248, 249
Silicic acid process 82
Silybum marianum 240
Skin ulcerations 52
Smilax medica 251
Snapdragons 182
Snowball 126
Snowberry 126, 127
Soap wort 118
Solanaceae 243, 252
Solanum dulcamara 234
Solidago virgaurea 249
Soporific 51
Sound ether 15
Sowbread 235
Speedwell 184, 193
Spice cloves 163
Spurges 171, 244
Spurry 116
Squill 186
St. John's Worts 37
Stapelia 171
Starch 66
Starweeds 116
Sterculiaceae 178
Stinging nettle 90, 97
Stingless Nettle 251
Stitchworts 116
Stone ailments 248
Stone crops 171
Stone formation 249, 250
Stonecrop 51
Strawberries 125
Strophanthus 186, 210
Strophanthus hispidus 259
Strophanthus Species 214
Surinam cherry 163
Swamp birches 102
Sweet Flag 87
Sweet William 116
Sweet woodruff 250
Symphoricarpos racemosus 127
Syringa 201
Syzygeum aromaticum 163
Szygium jambolana 164

T
Tabasheer 82

Tannin 22, 40, 95, 102, 163, 167, 218
Taraxacum officinale 240
Tares 81
Terebinthineae 90
Teucrium scorodonia 254
Thuja 33
Thyroid gland swellings 62
Tiliaceae 178
Tin process 237
Tongue grass 116
Tonsillitis 59
Trace elements 73
Tropical trees and shrubs 91

U
Umbelliferae 248
Unsaturated fatty acid 135
Urine retention 249, 250
Urticales 90

V
Vaccinium Myrtillus 222
Vaccinium vitis idaea 222
Valerian 127
Verbascum Thapsiforme 192
Veronica agrestis 93
Veronica officinalis 193
Vetiver oil 75
Viburnum 126
Vines 210
Vitaceae 119
Vitamin A 111, 134
Vitamin A deficiency 229
Vitamin C 52, 110, 130
Vitamin D 187
Vitamins 137, 145
Vitis vinifera 120, 125
Volatile oils 30

W
Wall flower 186
Wall pepper 51
Walnut 91
Warmth ether 15, 59, 111, 155
Warmth organization 28
Water Pennywort 249
Wax myrtle 91
Weak thinking 59
Weigela 126
White bryony 56

White horehound 242
Willow 91, 102
Wine–rue..90
Wintergreen.................................102
Wood Sorrels 170
Wound healing 42

Y
Yarrow 97, 240
Yucca filamentosa 242

Z
Zantedeschia aethiopica 84